Contents

Preface

The aim of this book is to provide an introduction to the syndrome of diabetes mellitus. The emphasis is firmly on clinical aspects of diabetes although insights into aetiology and pathophysiology have been included wherever possible.

It is hoped that the book will be of interest to medical undergraduates and postgraduate examination candidates.

A. J. K.
1996

COLOUR GUIDE

Diabetes

Andrew J. K   MRCP

Consultant Physic   id Endo
Southampton Un
Southampton, UK

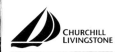

CHURCHILL
LIVINGSTONE

NEW YORK EDINBURGH LONDON MADRID MELBOURNE SAN FRANCISCO
AND TOKYO 1997

CHURCHILL LIVINGSTONE
Medical Division of Pearson Professional Limited

Distributed in the United States of America by Churchill
Livingstone Inc., 650 Avenue of the Americas, New York,
N.Y. 10011, and by associated companies, branches and
representatives throughout the world.

First published 1997

ISBN 0-443-05080-5

British Library Cataloguing in Publication Data
A catalogue record for this book is available from the
British Library

Library of Congress Cataloging in Publication Data
A catalog record for this book is available from the Library
of Congress

Medical knowledge is constantly changing. As new
information becomes available, changes in treatment,
procedures, equipment and the use of drugs become
necessary. The author and the publishers have, as far
as it is possible, taken care to ensure that the
information given in the text is accurate and up to
date. However, readers are strongly advised to confirm
that the information, especially with regard to drug
usage, complies with current legislation and standards
of practice.

For Churchill Livingstone:
Publisher: Michael Parkinson
Project Editors: Jim Kilgore, Janice Urquhart
  Copy Editor: Adam Campbell
  Indexer: Helen McKillop
Project Controller: Nancy Arnott

Printed in Hong Kong

Acknowledgements

The slide collection of the Diabetic Clinic, The General Hospital, Birmingham, formed the basis of this book. The collection was established under the supervision of Dr M. G. Fitzgerald, Dr M. Nattrass, Dr A. D. Wright and the late Professor J. Malins. The author gratefully acknowledges all the departmental staff who contributed to the collection. In addition, I would like to thank the following friends and colleagues for generous contributions from their own slide collections: Ms G. Hegarty (Fig. 2), Dr P. Gallagher (Figs 4, 99, 100, 106, 107, and 121), Dr A. Foulis (Fig. 15), Professor G. F. Bottazzo (Fig. 18), Dr A. Clarke (Fig. 19), Dr D. I. Phillips (Fig. 20), Dr C. J. Bailey (Figs 21 and 45), Dr S. O'Rahilly (Fig. 37), Professor E. J. Thomas (Fig. 39), Dr X. Khader (Fig. 82), Dr R. E. J. Ryder (Figs 85 and 86), Dr P. Newrick (Fig. 87), Dr A. J. Howie (Fig. 92), Dr M. Rogerson (Fig. 94), Mr A. R. Ready (Fig. 95), Mr N. J. M. London (Figs 96, 97 and 98), Dr A. M. Davies (Fig. 116), Dr I. A. MacFarlane (Fig. 123), Dr B. A. Leatherdale (Fig. 124), Dr J. A. Edge (Fig. 125) and Professor A. J. Sinclair (Fig. 126).

Thanks also go to: Clinical Illustration and Information Design, The Dental Hospital, Birmingham; The Department of Medical Illustration, The General Hospital, Birmingham; Teaching Support and Media Services, Southampton University Hospitals; the staff of the Diabetes Resource Centre, The General Hospital, Birmingham, UK.

Figs 5–8 are reproduced courtesy of The Photographic Library, The Wellcome Centre for Clinical Science; Fig. 10 (Green S et al 1992 Incidence of childhood-onset insulin-dependent diabetes mellitus: the EURODIAB ACE study. Lancet 339: 905–909), is reproduced by permission of the Lancet; Fig. 63 (Meeking D R, Krentz A J Pneumomediastinum complicating diabetic ketoacidosis. Diabetic Medicine, in press), is reproduced with permission of John Wiley & Sons Ltd; Fig. 115 (Krentz A J et al 1989 Journal of the Royal College of Physicians of London 23: 111–113) is reproduced with permission of the Royal College of Physicians of London; Fig. 122 (Rupp M E 1995 Rhinocerebral mucormycosis. New England Journal of Medicine 33: 564) is reprinted by permission of the Massachusetts Medical Society; Fig. 123 (Eyes B, MacFarlane I A 1986 Radiology of diabetes. MTP Press, Lancaster) is reproduced with permission of the authors and publishers.

1 / The syndrome of diabetes mellitus

Definition

Diabetes mellitus is a syndrome – i.e. a collection of disorders – characterized by defective regulation of multiple aspects of carbohydrate, lipid and protein metabolism. The biochemical hallmark of diabetes mellitus is chronic hyperglycaemia.

Clinical presentation

The myriad clinical manifestations of diabetes mellitus range from asymptomatic cases of non-insulin-dependent diabetes to the dramatic life-threatening syndromes of diabetic ketoacidosis and hyperosmolar non-ketosis (see pp. 43–46). Non-insulin-dependent diabetes may also present with chronic micro- or macrovascular complications.

Chronic complications of diabetes

Microvascular disease. While the acute osmotic symptoms of diabetes can usually be controlled with appropriate therapy, diabetes is also associated with the insidious development of specific multi-organ damage primarily affecting the retina (Fig. 1, see pp. 47–52), renal glomerulus (Fig. 2, see pp. 63–64) and peripheral nervous system (see pp. 55–62). These tissues are freely permeable to glucose, and the small-vessel (microvascular) complications of diabetes are closely linked to glycaemic control. The ultimate clinical sequelae of diabetic microvascular disease include blindness, end-stage renal failure (Fig. 2), foot ulceration and gangrene (Fig. 3).

Macrovascular disease. Diabetes is also associated with an increased mortality from atherosclerotic complications, particularly myocardial infarction (Fig. 4, see pp. 71–72). These metabolic and vascular complications are major causes of morbidity and mortality on a global scale.

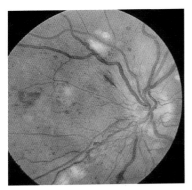

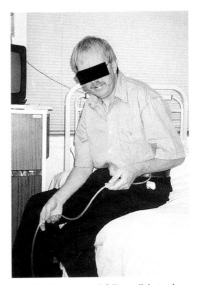

Fig. 1 Diabetic retinopathy is the leading cause of blindness under the age of 65 in the UK.

Fig. 2 End-stage renal failure; diabetes is now the commonest cause in western countries.

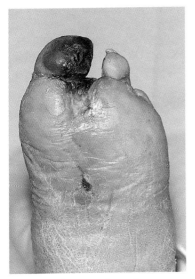

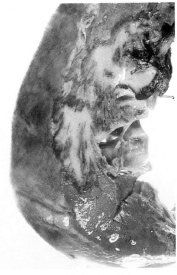

Fig. 3 Diabetic neuropathy confers a greatly increased risk of gangrene and amputation.

Fig. 4 Myocardial infarction; diabetes mellitus is a major risk factor for atherosclerosis.

2 / A brief history

The pre-insulin era

The Egyptians described clinical states of polyuria as long ago as 1550 BC (Fig. 5). Aretaeus of Cappadocia (2nd century AD) is credited with the earliest use of the term 'diabetes' (Greek: a siphon). The link with disordered carbohydrate metabolism was made by physicians in India (c. 500–600 AD) who found that the urine of diabetic patients 'tasted like honey' and attracted ants. In the 18th century, Matthew Dobson of Liverpool demonstrated that the urine from diabetic patients contained sugar and that the serum tasted sweet. A contemporary of Dobson's, John Rollo, was one of the first physicians to use the adjective 'mellitus' (from the Latin 'sweet') to distinguish the condition from other states of polyuria ('insipidus') not attributable to glycosuria. Claude Bernard (1813–1878) demonstrated the storage of glycogen in the liver and the induction of '*piqûre*' diabetes in the rabbit. In 1869, a Berlin medical student, Paul Langerhans (1847–1888), described the eponymous clusters ('islets') of endocrine cells in the pancreas (Fig. 6). In 1874, Professor Adolf Kussmaul of Freiburg University (1822–1902) described the 'air hunger' of ketoacidosis. In 1889, Oskar Minkowski (Fig. 7) and Josef Von Mering in Strasbourg noted the appearance of glycosuria and hyperglycaemia following pancreatectomy in a dog. The Belgian physician Jean de Meyer coined the word 'insulin' (Latin: island) in 1909.

The discovery of insulin

During 1921–1922, Frederick Banting, Charles Best, James Collip and Professor J. J. R. Macleod at the University of Toronto isolated pancreatic extracts suitable for clinical use (Fig. 8). On 11 January 1922, Leonard Thompson, aged 14 years, was the first diabetic patient to receive insulin.

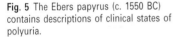

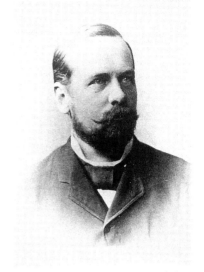

Fig. 5 The Ebers papyrus (c. 1550 BC) contains descriptions of clinical states of polyuria.

Fig. 6 Paul Langerhans – insulin-producing B-cells form the major endocrine component of the islets.

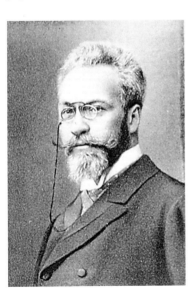

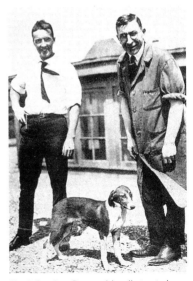

Fig. 7 Oskar Minkowski (1858–1931) – physician and scientist.

Fig. 8 Banting, Best and insulin-treated pancreatectomized dog – University of Toronto, 1922.

3 / Classification of diabetes mellitus

Diabetes mellitus

In 1980, the World Health Organization proposed a classification of diabetes mellitus based on recommendations of the US National Diabetes Data Group. The classification, revised in 1985, has been accepted internationally (Fig. 9). Of the main subtypes, insulin-dependent diabetes mellitus (IDDM or type 1 diabetes) is characterized by the development of ketoacidosis and the reliance on exogenous insulin (see pp. 11–14). On a global basis, however, non-insulin-dependent diabetes mellitus (NIDDM or type 2 diabetes) is the most prevalent form (see pp. 15–16). Diabetes is associated with many genetic and acquired syndromes (see pp. 17–22) and drugs (see p. 17).

Impaired glucose tolerance

The 1980 WHO classification introduced the intermediate diagnostic category of impaired glucose tolerance which replaced poorly defined entities such as 'chemical diabetes'. The introduction of this category recognized an area of diagnostic uncertainty between normality and diabetes, in which patients are not at risk of developing the microvascular complications of diabetes. However, impaired glucose tolerance carries a relatively high risk of progression to diabetes mellitus and confers some of the increased risk of macrovascular disease associated with diabetes. The diagnosis can only be made on a 75 g oral glucose tolerance test; fasting blood glucose concentration (venous plasma) must be <7.8 mmol/l with a 2 h level between 7.8 and 11.1 mmol/l (Fig. 14, p. 10). The diagnostic criteria vary according to the blood sample, the corresponding levels being 8.9–12.2 mmol/l for capillary plasma.

A. CLINICAL CLASSES

Diabetes mellitus
- Insulin-dependent diabetes mellitus (Type 1; IDDM)
- Non-insulin-dependent diabetes mellitus (Type 2; NIDDM)
    (a) non-obese
    (b) obese
- Malnutrition-related diabetes mellitus
- Other types of diabetes mellitus associated with certain conditions and syndromes
    (1) pancreatic disease causing diabetes
    (2) diabetes due to other endocrine disease
    (3) drug or toxin-induced diabetes
    (4) abnormalities of insulin or its receptors
    (5) diabetes associated with genetic syndromes
    (6) miscellaneous causes of diabetes
- Gestational diabetes mellitus
- Impaired glucose tolerance
    (a) non-obese
    (b) obese
    (c) associated with certain conditions and syndromes

B. STATISTICAL RISK CLASSES

- Previous abnormality of glucose tolerance
- Potential abnormality of glucose tolerance

Fig. 9 WHO (1985) classification of diabetes and allied categories of glucose intolerance (Reference – Diabetes mellitus. Report of a study group (Technical Report Series 727). World Health Organization, Geneva, 1985).

4 / Epidemiology of diabetes mellitus

Insulin-dependent diabetes

The incidence of insulin-dependent diabetes mellitus shows considerable geographic variation. The highest rates are in Finland (>30 cases/year per 100 000 population), Norway, Sweden and Denmark (Fig. 10), with Japan having the lowest incidence amongst developed countries. A high incidence in Sardinia contrasts with the low incidence in the rest of the Mediterranean. In some countries, e.g. Finland, Poland and Scotland, the incidence has been increasing. Variable incidence rates between and within populations are cited as evidence of pathogenic effects of environmental factors (e.g. viruses; see p. 11).

Non-insulin-dependent diabetes

Prevalence rates vary markedly between populations. Non-insulin-dependent diabetes accounts for >85% of diabetes in the UK (see p. 15). The prevalence increases with age, with up to 20% of the over-80s being affected. This form of diabetes also accounts for the majority of cases in developing countries. The highest prevalence rates (up to 35% of adults) occur in populations that have undergone radical changes from traditional to 'Westernized' lifestyles (e.g. North American Indians, Pacific Islanders, Australian Aborigines). The Pima Indians of Arizona have the highest recorded prevalence with over 50% of adults aged 35 years or older having diabetes (Fig. 11). The 'Thrifty Genotype' hypothesis (of Neel) proposes that these populations have genetic traits that once conferred survival advantages but which have been rendered detrimental by abundant food supplies. The prevalence of diabetes is also high in migrant populations, e.g. south Asians in the UK have an incidence rate four times that of the indigenous white population (Fig. 12).

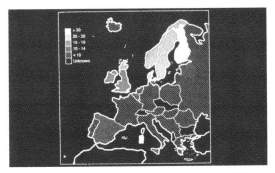

Fig. 10 Age-standardized childhood incidence (per 100 000 per year) of insulin-dependent diabetes.

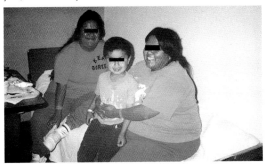

Fig. 11 The Pima Indians of Arizona have the highest prevalence of diabetes in the world.

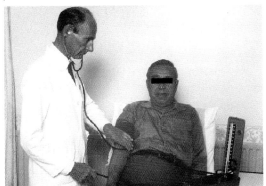

Fig. 12 South Asians in the UK have a high prevalence of diabetes and coronary heart disease.

5 / **Diagnosis of diabetes mellitus**

The diagnosis of diabetes mellitus relies upon the demonstration of chronic hyperglycaemia, as defined by the WHO diagnostic criteria. Diabetes cannot be diagnosed on the basis of glycosuria alone (Fig. 13), nor should the diagnosis rely upon indices of long-term glycaemia such as glycated haemoglobin or fructosamine.

Random plasma glucose

In patients presenting with typical symptoms (polyuria, polydipsia, weight loss despite maintenance of caloric intake, fatigue, drowsiness or coma), a single random measurement of circulating glucose is usually diagnostic (i.e. venous plasma glucose ≥11.1 mmol/l). In the absence of symptoms the diagnosis should be confirmed by a second blood glucose measurement.

Fasting plasma glucose

Following a 10 h overnight fast, a venous plasma glucose ≥7.8 mmol/l is diagnostic of diabetes. Levels below this are compatible with normality or impaired glucose tolerance.

Oral glucose test

A 75 g oral glucose tolerance test, performed under standardized conditions, is rarely necessary for the diagnosis of diabetes. The main indications for a glucose tolerance test are:

- non-diagnostic blood glucose concentrations
- diagnosis of gestational diabetes mellitus
- diagnosis of impaired glucose tolerance
- confirmation of a low renal threshold for glucose (i.e. <10 mmol/l; Fig. 14).

N.B. – glucose tolerance testing is contraindicated in patients with marked hyperglycaemia, in whom the test is, in any case, unnecessary.

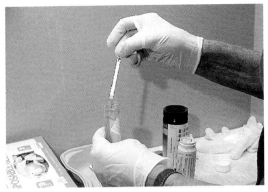

Fig. 13 Although useful in case-finding, diabetes cannot be diagnosed using urine tests for glucose.

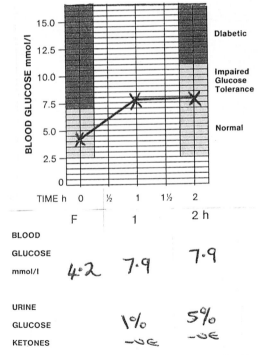

Fig. 14 Low renal threshold for glucose (5% glycosuria with blood glucose levels <10 mmol/l).

6 / Insulin-dependent diabetes mellitus

Pathophysiology   Insulin-dependent diabetes is characterized by autoimmune-mediated selective destruction of the insulin-producing B-cells of the pancreatic islets in genetically predisposed individuals (Fig. 15). As a consequence, patients are completely reliant upon exogenous insulin to prevent ketosis and thereby preserve life (Fig. 16). Plasma levels of C-peptide (a marker of endogenous insulin secretion) are undetectable in established insulin-dependent diabetes. However, C-peptide concentrations are not measured routinely in clinical practice.

Genetic factors   Class II major histocompatibility complex (MHC) genes on the short arm of chromosome 6 are responsible for most of the genetic susceptibility to the disease, with 95% of patients being positive for human-lymphocyte-associated (HLA) antigens DR3 or DR4 (compared with 40% of controls). The highest risk is in DR3/DR4 heterozygotes, whereas DR2 is protective. Certain DQ alleles are more common amongst patients with insulin-dependent diabetes. In addition, non-MHC genes (e.g. the insulin gene on the short arm of chromosome 11) modify risk.

Environmental factors   In monozygotic twins the concordance rate for the disease is only 30–50%, pointing to factors other than those inherited from parents. Putative environmental factors implicated in the aetiopathogenesis of insulin-dependent diabetes include viruses (rubella, coxsackie B4, cytomegalovirus) and certain foods (exposure to cows' milk in infancy, smoked products containing nitrosamines). To date, however, no precipitating environmental factor has been identified with certainty.

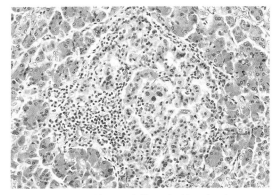

Fig. 15 Insulitis: the islets are infiltrated with a chronic inflammatory cell response.

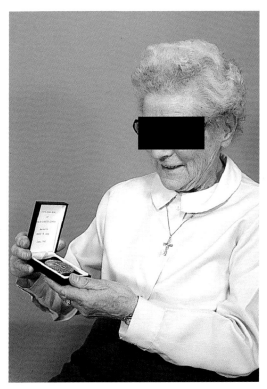

Fig. 16 UK patients treated with insulin for over 50 years are eligible for the Alan Nabarro medal.

Presenting The age of peak incidence is between 11 and 13
features years. The majority of patients are diagnosed before
the age of 30 years, although the disease may present
at any age, even in the elderly. A seasonal variation is
recognized, the incidence in older children and
adolescents being lowest during the summer.
Presentation is usually acute, with marked symptoms
and loss of body weight (Fig. 17). Ketonuria is
indicative of profound insulin deficiency. Ten percent
of patients present in ketoacidosis (see pp. 43 & 44).
Microvascular complications at diagnosis are
exceptionally rare.

Autoimmune Although the clinical presentation is usually abrupt,
markers prospective studies have demonstrated a preclinical
prodrome of several years. During this time,
autoimmune destruction of the islet B-cells is
occurring but symptoms appear only when >90% of
the insulin-producing cells are destroyed. Attempts at
limiting the final stages of B-cell destruction using
cyclosporin have met with only partial success.
Cytoplasmic islet cell antibodies are present in the
plasma of approximately 80% of patients at diagnosis
(Fig. 18). Family studies have shown that siblings of
an affected individual who are positive for these
antibodies are at an increased risk of developing the
disease, although this is not invariable. Antibodies
directed against insulin and the 64 kD islet antigen
glutamic acid decarboxylase may also be detectable.
These markers are not usually required for diagnosis
but are being utilized to identify high-risk subjects for
primary prevention studies.

Treatment With few exceptions, insulin is a life-long requirement
(see p. 45). A temporary partial remission or
'honeymoon period' may occur, when glycaemic
control is excellent with small doses of insulin.

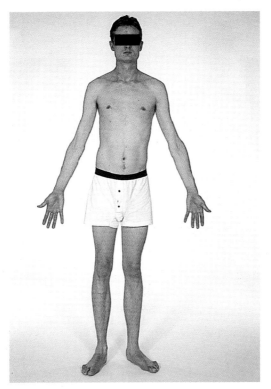

Fig. 17 Acute symptoms and pronounced weight loss are characteristic presenting features of IDDM.

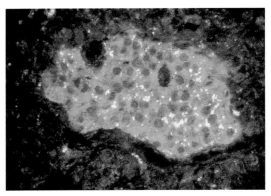

Fig. 18 Islet cell antibodies detected by indirect immunofluorescence on a human pancreas.

7 / Non-insulin-dependent diabetes mellitus

Pathogenesis   Patients with non-insulin-dependent diabetes secrete enough insulin to prevent ketosis but metabolism is not normalized. A 30–40% reduction in insulin-mediated glucose disposal leads to progressive compensatory fasting hyperinsulinaemia until fasting plasma glucose exceeds ~7 mmol/l. Islet mass is reduced with deposition of islet amyloid polypeptide (Fig. 19). Increased plasma levels of proinsulin-like molecules indicate B-cell dysfunction. The high concordance rate for identical twins (~90%) is cited as evidence of either a strong genetic component (generally non-HLA linked, cf. insulin-dependent diabetes) or a shared predisposing intrauterine environment (the 'Barker–Hales' hypothesis; Fig. 20). The disorder is clinically and biochemically heterogeneous. Obesity is common (75%) and is a prominent feature of some animal models, such as the *ob/ob* mouse which is deficient in an adipocyte-derived satiety-promoting protein (Fig. 21). Abdominal fat (Fig. 41, p. 28) is particularly associated with non-insulin-dependent diabetes. Transient gestational diabetes (see p. 81) is also a risk factor for the subsequent development of non-insulin-dependent diabetes.

Clinical features   Patients are usually over 40 years of age at diagnosis. A family history is common. A distinct subgroup ('maturity-onset diabetes of the young', MODY) is well-recognized (see p. 21). Presentation of non-insulin-dependent diabetes is usually with typical symptoms of diabetes, but many asymptomatic cases are diagnosed at screening or after presentation with associated disorders (e.g. myocardial infarction). Since the disease is often subclinical for many years, chronic microvascular complications (e.g. retinopathy, see pp. 47–52) are frequently present at diagnosis.

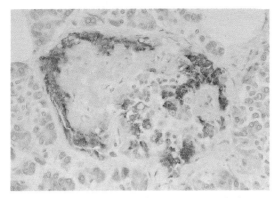

Fig. 19 Islet in NIDDM – reduced insulin content (stained brown) and amyloid deposits (Congo red stain).

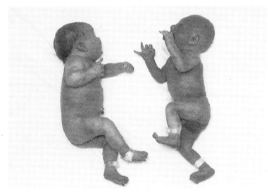

Fig. 20 The baby on the right has a lower ponderal index (weight/length^3) and a higher risk of NIDDM in adult life.

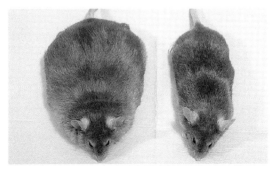

Fig. 21 An obese insulin-resistant, leptin-deficient diabetic ob/ob mouse and a homozygous (+/+) lean litter mate.

8 / Secondary diabetes mellitus

Diabetes mellitus may arise secondary to a number of hereditary and acquired diseases and as a consequence of certain drugs.

Pancreatic disease

Chronic pancreatitis is frequently complicated by glucose intolerance or diabetes (Fig. 22). Associated glucagon deficiency may contribute to severe hypoglycaemia in insulin-treated patients. Carcinoma of the pancreas is more common in patients with pre-existing diabetes and should be suspected in elderly patients presenting with weight loss, abdominal pain or obstructive jaundice. Diabetes developing *de novo* with pancreatic carcinoma is associated with insulin resistance (see p. 23) rather than insulinopenia. Pancreatectomy (>90%) necessitates life-long insulin therapy (Fig. 23). Diabetes may complicate cystic fibrosis, especially disease of long duration. Haemochromatosis is characterized by excessive iron deposition in a number of organs, with diabetes occurring in ~50% of cases (Figs 24 and 25). Fibrocalculous diabetes is a ketosis-resistant subtype of malnutrition-related diabetes mellitus encountered in the tropics.

Drugs

Many drugs may lead to the development of glucose intolerance or to a deterioration in glycaemic control in patients with pre-existing diabetes. Insulin resistance and/or impairment of endogenous insulin secretion have been implicated. Commonly encountered examples include:

- corticosteroids (especially high doses)
- diuretics (thiazide, loop and potassium-sparing)
- beta-blockers (especially non-selective agents)
- beta-adrenergic agonists (especially parenteral)
- cyclosporin A (e.g. renal transplant recipients).

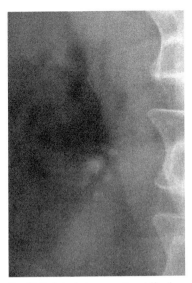

Fig. 22 Radiological pancreatic calcification in a patient with chronic pancreatitis and diabetes.

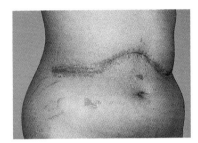

Fig. 23 Total pancreatectomy (here for painful chronic pancreatitis) necessitates insulin therapy.

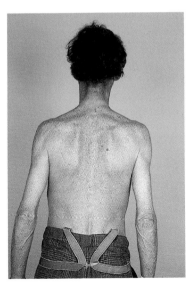

Fig. 24 Haemochromatosis: the classic 'bronzed' pigmentation is due to tissue iron deposition.

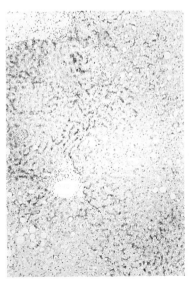

Fig. 25 Liver biopsy showing siderosis (Prussian blue reaction with Perls' reagent).

Endocrinopathies

Hypersecretion of hormones which antagonize the actions of insulin (i.e. counter-regulatory hormones) are associated with glucose intolerance and diabetes mellitus. Deteriorating glycaemic control may be the presenting feature of an endocrinopathy developing in a diabetic patient (see also p. 23). The most common of these is Graves' disease, an autoimmune form of thyrotoxicosis which is more prevalent in patients with insulin-dependent diabetes (Fig. 26). Other less common endocrinopathies include:

- acromegaly (30% have impaired glucose tolerance and 30% have diabetes mellitus; Fig. 27)
- Cushing's syndrome (especially due to ectopic ACTH secretion; Fig. 28)
- Conn's syndrome (glucose intolerance in ~50%)
- glucagonoma (rare; Fig. 34, p. 24)
- phaeochromocytoma (rare; Fig. 35, p. 24)
- somatostatinoma (very rare).

By contrast, hormonal deficiencies in the following autoimmune disorders may lead to a decrease in insulin requirements:

- primary hypothyroidism
- Addison's disease.

In addition, the development of hypopituitarism (low levels of growth hormone and cortisol; Fig. 29) will lead to increased insulin sensitivity.

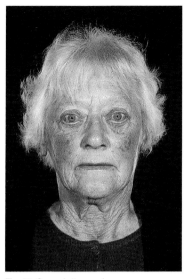

Fig. 26 Graves' disease is more common in patients with insulin-dependent diabetes.

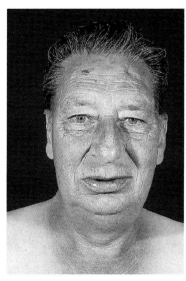

Fig. 27 Acromegaly is frequently associated with glucose intolerance or diabetes mellitus.

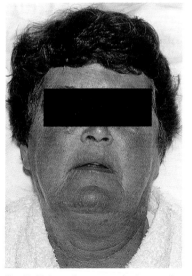

Fig. 28 Diabetes is common in the ectopic ACTH syndrome (here due to a bronchial carcinoma).

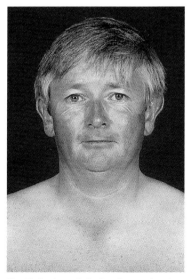

Fig. 29 Panhypopituitarism is associated with reduced insulin requirements in IDDM patients.

9 / Genetic syndromes associated with diabetes mellitus

Diabetes (mainly non-insulin-dependent) is associated with a number of inherited syndromes.

Chromosomal defects

These include Down's syndrome (trisomy or translocation of chromosome 21), Turner's syndrome (karyotype 45 XO; Fig. 30), Klinefelter's syndrome (47, XXY) and Prader-Willi syndrome (deletion/translocation of chromosome 15).

Neurodegenerative disorders

Myotonic dystrophy (Fig. 31) is an autosomal dominant multisystem disorder which is due to expansion of a trinucleotide repeat on chromosome 19. It is associated with insulin resistance but overt diabetes is relatively uncommon. Friedreich's ataxia (autosomal recessive) is associated with diabetes.

DIDMOAD (Wolfram) syndrome

This is a rare autosomal recessive syndrome comprising diabetes mellitus, diabetes insipidus, optic atrophy, nerve deafness and hydronephrosis presenting in childhood (Fig. 32).

Maturity-Onset Diabetes of the Young (MODY)

This uncommon form of non-insulin-dependent diabetes is a heterogeneous autosomal dominant disorder (Fig. 33) characterized by fasting hyperglycaemia and relative insulinopenia, which presents before the age of 25 years. Several distinct genetic subtypes have been identifed, including mutations in the gene encoding the B-cell glucose 'sensing' enzyme glucokinase.

Maternally-inherited diabetes

Syndromes associated with mitochondrial DNA mutations account for only a small proportion (<1% of non-insulin-dependent diabetes in the UK.

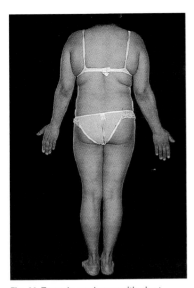

Fig. 30 Turner's syndrome with short stature and valgus – patient had insulin-treated diabetes.

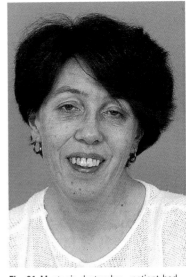

Fig. 31 Myotonic dystrophy – patient had normal glucose tolerance but marked hyperinsulinaemia.

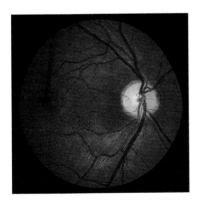

Fig. 32 Optic atrophy in the DIDMOAD syndrome.

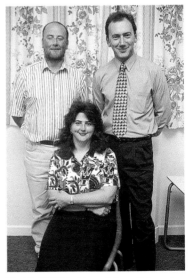

Fig. 33 MODY in three siblings (father also affected) – all well controlled by sulphonylureas.

10 / Biochemistry of diabetes mellitus

The chronic hyperglycaemia of diabetes reflects an absolute or relative deficiency of insulin and/or the hormone's tissue effects. Other key aspects of intermediary metabolism, including fat and protein, are also affected to variable degrees. Insulin's anabolic effects are antagonized by glucagon (Fig. 34), catecholamines (Fig. 35), growth hormone (Fig. 27, p. 20) and cortisol (Fig. 28, p. 20).

Insulin-dependent diabetes
In established insulin-dependent diabetes, endogenous insulin secretion is negligible. Plasma glucagon and catecholamine levels are elevated but return towards normal with insulin therapy. Insulin deficiency has major implications for fat and protein metabolism. Adipocyte lipolysis (the breakdown of triglyceride to non-esterified fatty acids and glycerol) is disinhibited, and fatty acids taken up by the liver are converted into ketone bodies. Ketonuria (in concert with hyperglycaemia) indicates marked insulin deficiency since lipolysis is inhibited at relatively low plasma insulin levels. Protein synthesis is decreased while breakdown of structural proteins contributes to loss o body weight.

Non-insulin-dependent diabetes
A relative deficiency of endogenous insulin in the presence of impaired insulin action leads to increased hepatic glucose production and decreased insulin-mediated glucose uptake by muscle (see p. 15).

Insulin resistance

This is defined as 'a reduced biological response to insulin'. The presence of insulin resistance is implied by normo- or hyperglycaemia in concert with hyperinsulinaemia. For research purposes, insulin action can be quantified using techniques such as the hyperinsulinaemic glucose 'clamp' (Fig. 36).

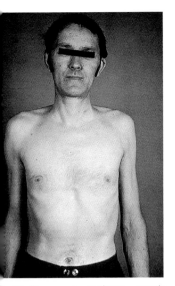

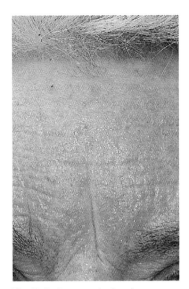

g. 34 Glucagonoma syndrome – muscle-
-asting and diabetes reflect the catabolic
fects of glucagon.

Fig. 35 Profuse perspiration due to
catecholamine excess in a patient with a
phaeochromocytoma.

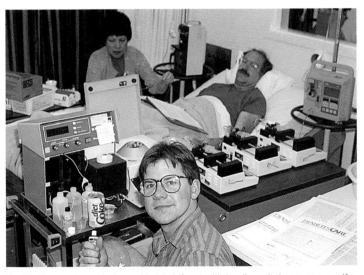

Fig. 36 Glucose clamp study – subject is infused with insulin and glucose to quantify
insulin action.

Clinical significance Insulin resistance is a major feature of non-insulin-dependent diabetes mellitus and appears to be an inherited metabolic defect. Obesity, which is common amongst patients with non-insulin-dependent diabetes, is also associated with insulin resistance, although in the absence of islet B-cell dysfunction, normal glucose tolerance is maintained.

Extreme insulin resistance

A number of rare syndromes are associated with defective cellular insulin receptor structure and function. The molecular biology of some of these syndromes, e.g. Leprechaunism (Fig. 37), Rabson-Mendenhall syndrome, has been elucidated. Severe insulin resistance may be accompanied by physical stigmata such as the dermatological condition acanthosis nigricans (Fig. 38). Polycystic ovary syndrome (Fig. 39) is a relatively common cause of insulin resistance which is associated with features of hyperandrogenism (hirsutism, amenorrhoea, etc.).

Lipoatrophic diabetes

This may be congenital or acquired and is characterized by partial or total absence of subcutaneous fat, variable degrees of insulin resistance and hyperlipidaemia (Fig. 40).

Syndrome X/Reaven's syndrome

Insulin resistance has been implicated in a number of pathological states which frequently co-segregate and which are associated with an increased risk of atherosclerotic disease. Key features include:

- decreased insulin-mediated glucose disposal
- glucose intolerance or diabetes mellitus
- hyperinsulinaemia
- elevated triglycerides and low HDL-cholesterol.
- essential hypertension
- abdominal (android) obesity.

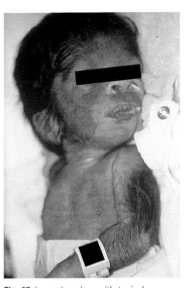

Fig. 37 Leprechaunism with typical features, including dysmorphic facies and hypertrichosis.

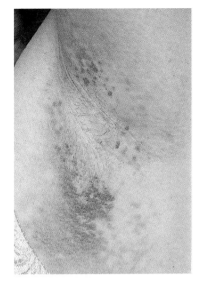

Fig. 38 Axillary acanthosis nigricans in a young woman with hyperinsulinaemia and glucose intolerance.

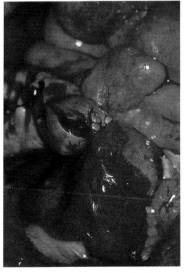

Fig. 39 Polycystic ovaries identified at laparotomy.

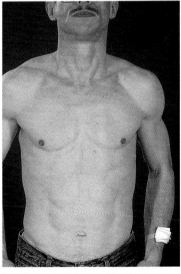

Fig. 40 Acquired lipoatrophic diabetes – marked hypertriglyceridaemia also present.

11 / Treatment: diet

Aims of diet
in diabetes
- To normalize glycaemia and blood lipids.
- To attain ideal body weight (Fig. 41).
- To minimize iatrogenic risks of hypoglycaemia.
- To achieve normal growth and development.
- To minimize macrovascular complications.

Obesity

Body mass index (BMI) is calculated by the formula: body weight (kg)/height (m^2). A BMI of ~20–25 is ideal. In the general population, mortality rates rise as body weight increases, particularly for BMI values >40. Obesity reduces insulin sensitivity (see pp. 15, 23 and 25).

Non-insulin-dependent diabetes
Key aspects of dietary advice include the following:

- reduce total energy intake if overweight or obese
- carbohydrate (principally as complex carbohydrate) should provide 50–55% of daily calorie requirements
- reduce fat intake to ~30% of total daily calories, with saturated fats supplying <10% total energy
- limit alcohol intake if overweight or hypertensive.

Teaching sessions involving relatives are useful adjuncts to dietary prescriptions. Special diabetic foods are unnecessary. The roles of anorectic drugs, very low-calorie diets and surgical procedures (e.g. gastric stapling, jaw wiring; Fig. 42) are limited.

Insulin-dependent diabetes
Regular intake of carbohydrate, including snacks between main meals, is usually necessary to avoid hypoglycaemia. Insulin-treated patients should always carry a readily available source of carbohydrate (e.g. glucose tablets) and should be educated (Fig. 43) about the dietary aspects of sport and exercise, travel and strategies for coping with intercurrent illnesses.

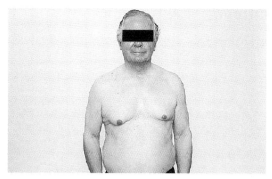

Fig. 41 Central obesity is more strongly associated with insulin resistance and NIDDM than lower body (gynoid) obesity.

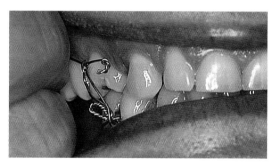

Fig. 42 Jaw wires may facilitate weight reduction but are generally a short-term measure.

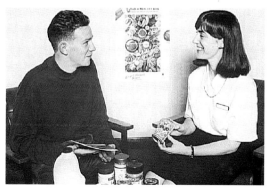

Fig. 43 Expert dietary advice is essential for diabetic patients.

12 / Treatment: sulphonylureas

Sulphonylureas are the principal oral agents used in patients with residual endogenous insulin secretion. 'First-generation' drugs (e.g. chlorpropamide, tolbutamide) have largely been superseded by more potent (on a molar basis) 'second-generation' drugs (e.g. glibenclamide, gliclazide), despite little difference in overall effectiveness.

Mode of action
The main pharmacological effect of sulphonylureas is the augmentation of insulin release from islet B-cells. The drugs bind to specific receptors, thereby inducing closure of ATP-sensitive potassium channels. Subsequent membrane depolarization leads to insulin secretion.

Indications
Sulphonylurea drugs are useful in patients with non-insulin-dependent diabetes who fail to respond adequately to dietary measures. A small proportion of patients will not respond to a sulphonylurea ('primary failures'), while insulin treatment also becomes necessary in 5–10% of patients per annum ('secondary failures') who respond initially.

Contra-indications
- Insulin-dependent diabetes mellitus.
- Pregnancy (insulin should be used if necessary).
- Peri-operatively (Fig. 44, see p. 41).

Adverse effects
Adverse effects are uncommon but include:

- Weight gain (due to hyperinsulinaemia).
- Hypoglycaemia. This is usually minor but rarely may be severe and protracted, especially in elderly patients treated with long-acting agents (see p. 39). Tolbutamide, gliclazide and glipizide are safer. The lowest dose should always be used initially.
- Alcohol-induced flushing (usually chlorpropamide).
- Hyponatraemia with chlorpropamide (in 5% of cases).
- Cutaneous hypersensitivity reactions (Fig. 45).

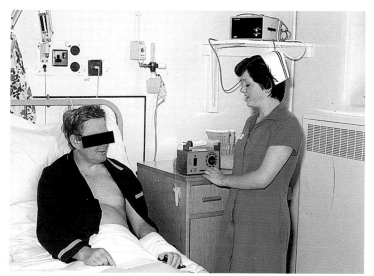

Fig. 44 Insulin should be used in preference to oral antidiabetic agents in patients undergoing major surgery.

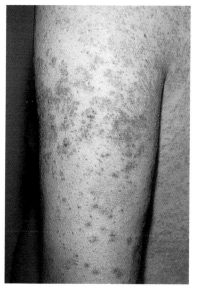

Fig. 45 Drug rashes (here due to glibenclamide) are uncommon, especially with 'second generation' agents.

13 / Treatment: metformin and other agents

Metformin

Metformin is the only biguanide available in the UK and the USA. Phenformin was withdrawn in the 1970s due to an unacceptable incidence of fatal lactic acidosis. Metformin does not stimulate endogenous insulin secretion but improves tissue insulin sensitivity (Fig. 46). It inhibits gluconeogenesis, thereby reducing hepatic glucose production. It is usually used in obese patients with non-insulin-dependent diabetes as an adjunct to diet. It does not cause hypoglycaemia when used as monotherapy. Metformin may be usefully combined with sulphonylureas although insulin may be required as NIDDM progresses. Metformin is associated with a relatively high frequency (up to 20% of patients) of unwanted effects, notably gastrointestinal disturbances. Patients who develop diarrhoea with metformin may undergo unnecessary investigations (Fig. 47). Lactic acidosis may ensue under conditions of (a) increased lactate production (e.g. tissue hypoxia) or (b) decreased lactate clearance (e.g. hepatic disease), or (c) when renal elimination of metformin is impaired. Metformin is therefore contraindicated in:

- renal impairment
- hepatic disease or alcoholism
- ischaemic heart disease, heart failure, sepsis.

Other agents

Alpha-glucosidase inhibitors (e.g. acarbose) and guar (a non-absorbable soluble fibre) reduce or retard gastrointestinal carbohydrate absorption. Acarbose, like metformin, also reduces plasma insulin concentrations. Gastrointestinal side-effects are common. Drugs to ameliorate insulin resistance (e.g. troglitazone) are under evaluation. Traditional plant remedies are also often used by south-Asian patients (Fig. 48).

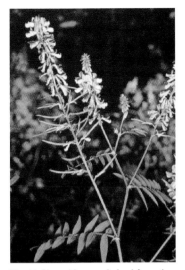

Fig. 46 Biguanides are derived from the traditional plant remedy *galega officinalis*.

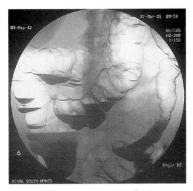

Fig. 47 Patients who develop diarrhoea due to metformin may undergo unnecessary radiology.

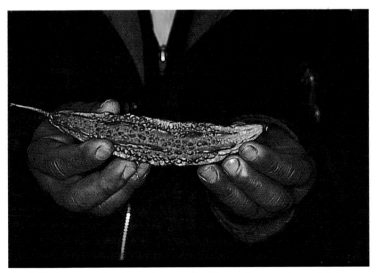

Fig. 48 Karela – a traditional hypoglycaemic plant that is often used by south-Asian diabetic patients.

14 / Treatment: insulin

Presently available insulin therapy falls short of physiological replacement for two reasons; first, subcutaneous insulin is delivered into the systemic rather than the portal circulation; secondly, plasma insulin profiles do not replicate normality. As a consequence, periods of relative over- and under-insulinization occur during the day and night. Glycaemic control is not normalized in most insulin-dependent patients, and the hazards of hypoglycaemia and ketoacidosis are ever present.

Preparations The main pharmacological preparations and their approximate durations of action are:

- soluble (4–6 hours)
- isophane (12–24 hours)
- lente (12–24 hours)
- ultralente (24–36 hours).

Most patients (>90%) are now treated with human sequence insulin manufactured by recombinant DNA techniques. No major differences in metabolic effects between porcine and human insulin have been observed, although the latter is less immunogenic (Figs 49 and 50). Genetically engineered insulin analogues with altered pharmacokinetics represent a novel therapeutic approach.

Delivery Most patients self-administer subcutaneous insulin between one and four times a day. Pre-mixed insulin (usually twice daily) in various fixed ratios of soluble: isophane (e.g. 30:70, 50:50) are popular and can be delivered using convenient pen injectors (Fig. 51). Multiple daily injections (soluble pre-meals, isophane at bedtime) are particularly suitable for younger patients. The long-term benefits of 'intensive' insulin therapy using multiple daily injections (or, less often, continuous subcutaneous infusion) are now recognized for carefully selected adults, but expertise is required for success and safety.

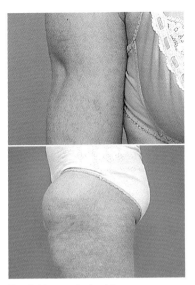

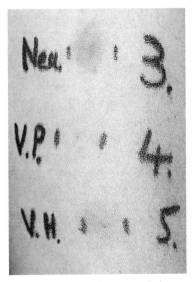

Fig. 49 Lipoatrophy (top) is uncommon; lipo-hypertrophy (bottom) reflects local lipogenesis.

Fig. 50 'Insulin allergy' may actually be a reaction to preservatives such as m-cresol.

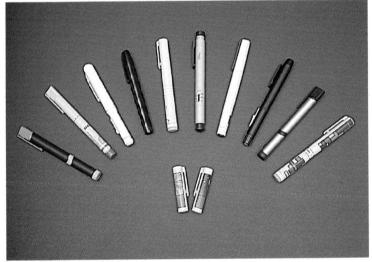

Fig. 51 Examples of some modern 'pen' injectors including disposable devices.

15 / **Monitoring metabolic control**

Urine tests

Urine tests using reagent-impregnated strips (see Fig. 13) can only provide a retrospective semi-quantitative indication of glycaemic control and may be misleading in elderly patients with high renal thresholds, i.e. >10 mmol/l (see p. 9). Furthermore, hypoglycaemia cannot be detected. Semi-quantitative test strips for acetocetate (e.g. Ketostix®) are also available for patients with insulin-dependent diabetes (see p. 43).

Home blood glucose tests

Self-testing of capillary blood glucose obtained by fingerprick (Fig. 52) is an established method for monitoring glycaemic control. Enzyme-impregnated strip methods are available which can be used in conjunction with reflectance meters to improve accuracy (Fig. 53). Specific meters are available for the visually impaired. Correct technique is a prerequisite for reliable readings.

Glycated haemoglobin

Haemoglobin A_{1c} is formed by the non-enzymatic glycation of the N-terminal valine residue of the β-chain of haemoglobin. The proportion of haemoglobin glycated to HbA_{1c} (normally approximately 4–6%) provides a clinically useful index of average glycaemia over the preceding 6–8 weeks. Spurious HbA_{1c} levels may arise in states of:

- blood loss/haemolysis (low HbA_{1c})
- elevated levels of HbS (low HbA_{1c})
- elevated levels of HbF (high HbA_{1c}).

Fructosamine

Fructosamine assays measure glycated plasma proteins, reflecting average glycaemia over the preceding 2–3 weeks. Levels can be misleading in hypoalbuminaemic states (Fig. 93, p. 64).

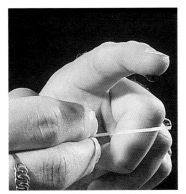

Fig. 52 Fingerprick testing of blood glucose using a glucose–oxidase test strip.

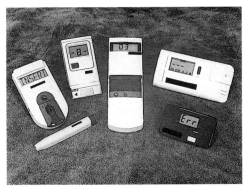

Fig. 53 Meters improve the accuracy of blood glucose monitoring – some can store results.

16 / Hypoglycaemia

Iatrogenic hypoglycaemia is the most serious hazard the treatment of diabetes mellitus. The great majority of episodes occur in insulin-treated patients, 10% of whom will experience, on average, one severe episode (i.e. causing coma or convulsions) per year. Severe hypoglycaemia complicating sulphonylurea therapy is uncommon but carries a relatively high (10%) mortality.

Aetiology   Hypoglycaemia in diabetic patients results from:

- a mismatch of glucose supply (e.g. a missed meal) and utilization (e.g. by physical exercise)
- a relative excess of insulin (either injected or stimulated by a sulphonylurea drug).

Clinical features   Cerebral function is vitally dependent on an adequate supply of glucose from the circulation. Accordingly, the most serious consequence of acute hypoglycaemia is cerebral dysfunction with the risk of coma (Fig. 54). Cognitive impairment progresses ultimately to loss of consciousness as blood glucose falls. Seizures and transient focal neurological deficits may occur. Prolonged severe hypoglycaemia, often exacerbated by excessive alcohol consumption, may produce cerebral oedema and permanent brain damage.

Warning symptoms   The onset of insulin-induced hypoglycaemia is usually heralded by symptoms of autonomic nervous system activation, e.g. tremor, sweating, anxiety, palpitations. If these warning symptoms are deficient or their perception is impaired (e.g. by certain drugs or alcohol) then the patient may become irrational and aggressive due to neuroglycopenia. Prompt assistance from another person may then be required to avert loss of consciousness and serious sequelae, including physical injury (Fig. 55).

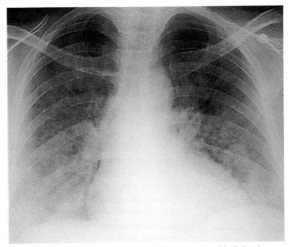

Fig. 54 Radiograph showing aspiration pneumonitis following insulin-induced hypoglycaemic coma.

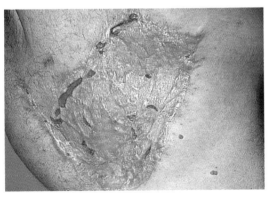

Fig. 55 Burn sustained following hypoglycaemia-induced coma in an insulin-treated patient.

Unrecognized hypoglycaemia

Long-term insulin treatment is associated with defective glucagon responses to hypoglycaemia. In addition, intensive insulin therapy (aiming for sustained near-normoglycaemia) may be associated with loss of autonomic hypoglycaemic warning symptoms, resulting in a high risk of recurrent severe hypoglycaemia. Antecedent hypoglycaemia appears to alter the glycaemic threshold for counter-regulatory hormone secretion; scrupulous avoidance of hypoglycaemia may restore symptoms. Unrecognized nocturnal hypoglycaemia is common and has been implicated in the sudden death of a few young patients ('dead in bed' syndrome).

Sulphonylureas and hypoglycaemia

Elderly patients are at risk of severe hypoglycaemia, particularly with longer-acting hypoglycaemia agents (e.g. chloropropamide, glibenclamide), and especially in circumstances of reduced caloric intake (e.g. during intercurrent illness). Agents predominantly excreted via the kidney (e.g. glibenclamide) should be avoided in renal impairment. Patients with severe sulphonylurea-induced hypoglycaemia should be admitted to hospital, since relapse following initial resuscitation with oral or intravenous glucose may necessitate prolonged infusions of glucose (Fig. 56). Diazoxide and octreotide inhibit endogenous insulin secretion and have been used as adjuncts to glucose.

Spontaneous hypoglycaemia

Insulin-secreting adenomas of the B-cells (insulinomas) are rare and have never been described in an insulin-dependent diabetic with hypoglycaemia (Fig. 57).

'Brittle' diabetes

This is a well-recognized cause of recurrent hypoglycaemia (see p. 83).

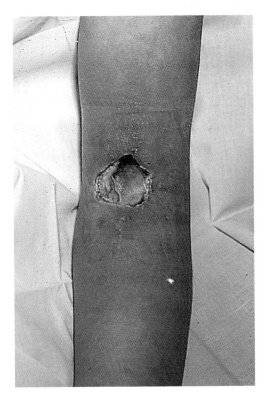

Fig. 56 Extravasation of 50% dextrose may cause tissue necrosis – a large vein should be cannulated.

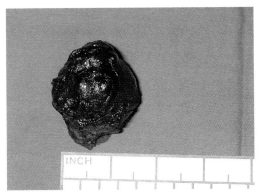

Fig. 57 Pancreatic insulinomas are a rare cause of spontaneous hypoglycaemia in non-diabetic patients.

17 / Surgery and intercurrent illness

Diabetics are more likely to require surgical treatment than are non-diabetics, e.g. limb amputation (Fig. 58; see p. 61), and are also more likely to have concurrent disease (e.g. ischaemic heart disease, autonomic neuropathy) which may adversely affect outcome (pp. 59 and 71). The hormonal stress response induced by surgical trauma may cause metabolic decompensation, the resulting catabolic state compromising tissue repair and recovery. Fluid and electrolyte disturbances may also be compounded by uncontrolled diabetes.

Non-insulin-dependent diabetes

In well-controlled patients, omission of sulphonylureas on the morning of surgery and avoidance of glucose- and lactate-containing intravenous fluids may be sufficient for minor procedures. Blood glucose levels should be monitored pre- and postoperatively. Long-acting sulphonylureas (e.g. chlorpropamide) should be discontinued several days prior to surgery since they may cause serious postoperative hypoglycaemia; insulin should be substituted. Metformin should also be avoided peri-operatively because of the risk of lactic acidosis. For major surgery, management should be as for insulin-treated patients.

Insulin-treated patients

For all but the most trivial procedures, patients should be stabilized pre-operatively using intravenous infusions of dextrose and insulin. Short-acting insulin (10–15 U) is added to 1 l of 5% dextrose (with 20 mmol/l KCl) and infused at 250 ml/h or infused simultaneously with dextrose via an infusion pump (Fig. 59). The insulin infusion rate is carefully adjusted to maintain blood glucose between 5 and 10 mmol/l.

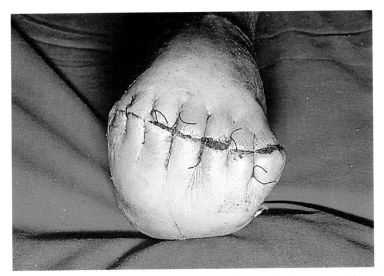

Fig. 58 Diabetic patients are at greatly increased risk of amputation for non-traumatic disease.

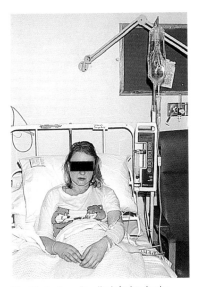

Fig. 59 Dextrose/insulin infusion in the management of a young patient with IDDM.

18 / Hyperglycaemic emergencies

Diabetic ketoacidosis

This usually affects younger insulin-dependent patients, in whom it remains a significant cause of morbidity and premature mortality. Ketoacidosis usually develops over hours or days in patients whose insulin dose is insufficient to counter the effects of markedly raised plasma counter-regulatory hormone levels. Infection is the most commonly identifiable cause of ketoacidosis.

Definition The cardinal biochemical features of DKA are:

- a metabolic acidosis (capillary or arterial bicarbonate 15 mmol/l or less) together with:

  (i) ketosis (urine Ketostix® reaction ++ or more)
  (ii) hyperglycaemia (with secondary dehydration and depletion of total body sodium and potassium.

Clinical features The patient is usually dehydrated and unwell with acidotic (Kussmaul) respiration. A depressed level of consciousness is associated with a worse prognosis. Other causes of coma must always be considered (Fig. 60). Signs of a precipitating cause may be evident (Fig. 61).

Diagnosis and management The diagnosis is confirmed by bedside tests of blood and urine. Urgent laboratory measurements of electrolytes (Fig. 62) and gases are essential. Management comprises:

- rehydration, initially with intravenous saline
- insulin (by continuous intravenous infusion)
- adequate replacement of potassium ions
- treatment of any precipitating cause.

The mortality rate is 5–10%, but is much higher (~50%) in the elderly. Complications include rhabdomyolysis, adult respiratory distress syndrome, cerebral oedema (especially in children; see Fig. 125, p. 84), rhinocerebral mucormycosis (Fig. 122, p. 80) and pneumomediastinum (Fig. 63).

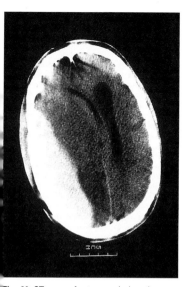

Fig. 60 CT scan of a trauma-induced extradural haematoma in a comatose ketoacidotic patient.

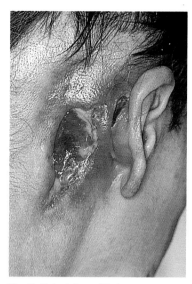

Fig. 61 Diabetic ketoacidosis was precipitated by this cutaneous abscess.

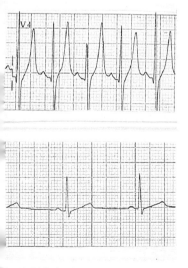

Fig. 62 ECG showing tachycardia and peaked T-waves of hyperkalaemia and response to treatment.

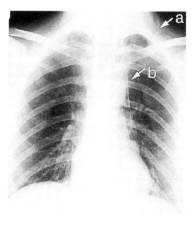

Fig. 63 Radiograph of surgical emphysema in neck tissues (a) and spontaneous pneumomediastinum (b).

Hyperosmolar non-ketotic coma

This is less common than ketoacidosis but carries a higher case-fatality rate. The syndrome usually develops in elderly patients with non-insulin-dependent diabetes and may be the presenting feature. Afro-Caribbeans are more likely to develop this syndome, this group accounting for approximately 25% of cases in the UK (Fig. 64). Certain drugs, notably beta-blockers and thiazide diuretics, have been implicated in the pathogenesis of the syndrome. Consumption of fizzy carbohydrate-containing drinks may exacerbate hyperglycaemia and dehydration.

Clinical features
The syndrome develops insidiously over a period of days with marked osmotic symptoms progressing to gradual clouding of consciousness (Fig. 65). Dehydration is usually profound with systemic hypotension. Coexisting and precipitating medical conditions are common. Focal neurological signs (Fig. 66), fits and coma may lead to an erroneous diagnosis of stroke. Acidosis is not a feature.

Diagnosis
There is marked hyperglycaemia (blood glucose usually >50 mmol/l) with dehydration and pre-renal uraemia; ketosis and acidosis are mild or absent. The plasma osmolality is elevated (to over 340 mmol/kg). Plasma osmolality is calculated as: 2 × (sodium + potassium) + urea + glucose.

Management
Fluid and insulin therapy is broadly similar to that for ketoacidosis (p. 43). Thromboembolic complications are frequent and these should be treated with anticoagulants. Although insulin is usually recommended for 2–3 months, black patients, in particular (including some presenting in DKA), may be well-controlled with sulphonylureas or diet alone (Fig. 64).

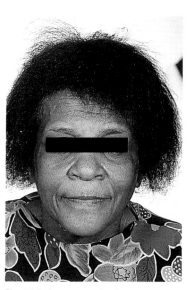

Fig. 64 Patients presenting in hyperosmolar coma may subsequently be controlled by sulphonylureas.

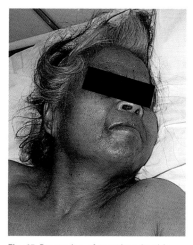

Fig. 65 Depression of conscious level is common in the hyperosmolar non-ketotic syndrome.

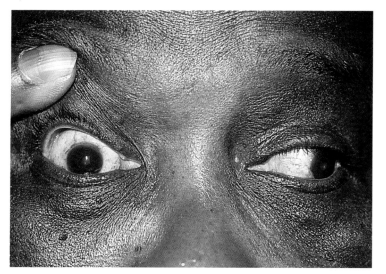

Fig. 66 Seizures or focal neurological signs may be mistaken for cerebrovascular events.

19 / **Diabetic retinopathy**

The principal factors determining the development of diabetic retinopathy are:

- duration of diabetes mellitus
- degree of chronic glycaemic control.

Classification   Diabetic retinopathy is classified as follows:

- background retinopathy (Fig. 67)
- pre-proliferative retinopathy (Fig. 68)
- proliferative retinopathy (Fig. 69)
- advanced diabetic eye disease
- maculopathy (see pp. 49–50).

Proliferative retinopathy and maculopathy are potentially sight-threatening forms of diabetic retinopathy. Advanced diabetic eye disease includes the sequelae of vitreous haemorrhage and secondary rubeotic glaucoma.

Insulin-dependent diabetes
Retinopathy is absent at diagnosis, but after 15 years of disease the prevalence is >95%. Up to 60% of patients develop sight-threatening proliferative retinopathy. The Diabetes Control and Complications Trial demonstrated a 76% reduction in the mean risk of developing retinopathy and a 54% reduction in the progression of pre-existing retinopathy in insulin-dependent patients treated with intensive insulin therapy. This reflected the ~2% lower HbA_{1c} levels in these patients. Retinopathy may deteriorate transiently following acute improvement in glycaemic control.

Non-insulin-dependent diabetes
Approximately 20% of patients have retinopathy at diagnosis, and careful fundoscopy is therefore mandatory in newly presenting patients. Maculopathy is the major cause of visual loss in this group of patients. This may, in part, reflect the additional effects of systemic hypertension.

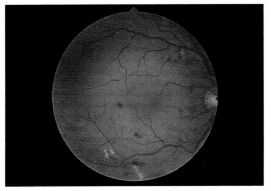

Fig. 67 Micro-aneurysms (dots), retinal haemorrhages (blots) and hard exudates.

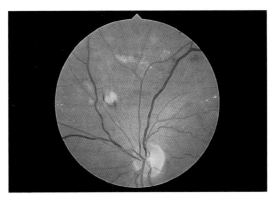

Fig. 68 Cotton wool spots are deep retinal infarcts which herald new vessel formation.

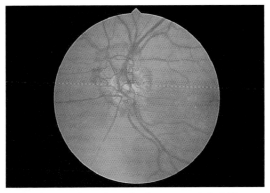

Fig. 69 New vessels on the optic disc are especially liable to bleed into the vitreous.

Background retinopathy
This is characterized opthalmoscopically by micro-aneurysms, intraretinal blot or flame haemorrhages and hard exudates (lipid deposits from leaking capillaries). These changes are usually asymptomatic.

Pre-proliferative retinopathy
Venous loops or beading and arterial sheathing with intraretinal microvascular abnormalities and cotton wool spots denote increasing retinal ischaemia.

Proliferative retinopathy
New vessels arise from the optic disc or periphery into areas of ischaemic retina. These friable vessels may cause pre-retinal (Fig. 70) or vitreous haemorrhages.

Advanced diabetic eye disease
Fibrous tissue associated with new vessels may cause traction and retinal detachment. Severe retinal ischaemia may lead to new vessel formation on the iris (Fig. 71). Obstruction of the angle by new vessel may cause painful secondary rubeotic glaucoma.

Maculopathy
Three types are recognized:

- exudative (Fig. 72)
- oedematous (cystic or diffuse – may be difficult to visualise on direct opthalmoscopy)
- ischaemic (the least amenable to treatment).

Maculopathy should be suspected if a significant reduction in visual acuity (i.e. by two lines on Snelle chart) occurs in the absence of an obvious cause suc as cataract formation. Slit lamp examination may be required to confirm the diagnosis. Leaking capillaries may be more easily identified by fluorescein angiography.

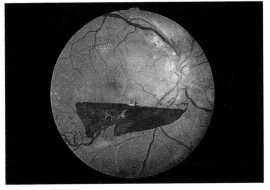

Fig. 70 Pre-retinal (subhyaloid) haemorrhages in a patient with diabetes and hypertension.

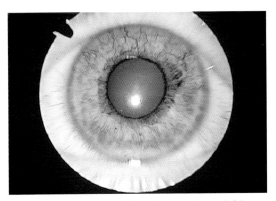

Fig. 71 New vessels on the iris causing secondary painful rubeotic glaucoma.

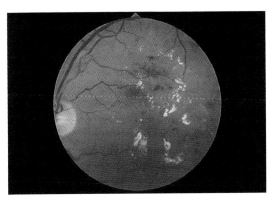

Fig. 72 Plaques of hard exudates at the macula threaten central vision.

Treatment **Laser therapy.** Timely laser therapy can reduce severe visual loss by >50% in patients with proliferative retinopathy or macular oedema. It is important that laser therapy is given before visual loss has become too severe and potentially irreversible. Laser therapy is an outpatient procedure. Several sittings may be necessary for extensive laser treatment which may involve thousands of retinal burns (Fig. 73). Night vision may be affected by extensive laser therapy.

Surgical vitrectomy. This specialized procedure may restore useful vision in selected patients with advanced diabetic eye disease. Microsurgical techniques are employed to remove fibrous plaques (Fig. 74), reattach areas of retina and apply intra-ocular laser if necessary.

Visual impairment
Patients with severe visual impairment should be registered partially sighted (corrected acuities 6/60) or blind (3/60, or worse), as appropriate. Low-vision aid and adapted everyday appliances are available.

Screening for diabetic retinopathy
Early recognition of diabetic retinopathy is crucial. Annual checks of corrected visual acuity combined with expert fundoscopy through pharmacologically dilated pupils is essential (Fig. 132, p. 88). Alternatively, non-mydriatic retinal cameras (Fig. 75) can provide colour photographs of the optic disc and macula. The photographs obtained using this technique require expert evaluation.

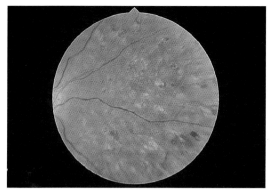

Fig. 73 Retinal scars from extensive laser therapy given for proliferative retinopathy.

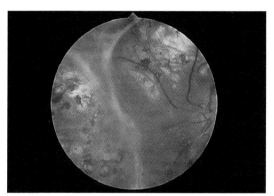

Fig. 74 Advanced diabetic eye disease with fibrous plaques may be amenable to surgical vitrectomy.

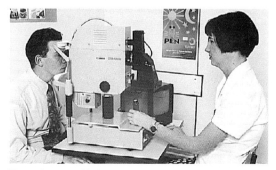

Fig. 75 A non-mydriatic camera – community-based screening requires a modifed van-housed camera.

20 / **Cataract**

Definition   A cataract is an opacity of the crystalline lens of the eye (Fig. 76). It may be asymptomatic in the early stages of development but may progress to cause significant visual impairment or even blindness. The commonest variety of cataract is the so-called 'senile cataract'. Cataracts are features of certain diseases and syndromes which may themselves be associated with diabetes, e.g. myotonic dystrophy (Fig. 31, p. 22).

Cataracts and diabetes   Epidemiological studies indicate that diabetes mellitus is a significant risk factor for cataract formation in patients aged up to 69 years. In patients in their 50s and 60s, the incidence of cataracts is 2–3 times greater than in the non-diabetic population. Rarely, diabetes is associated with the development of an acute form of rapidly developing lens opacity known as a 'snowflake cataract' (Fig. 77). This usually affects young insulin-dependent patients and typically, though not invariably, follows a period of particularly poor glycaemic control. The cataract may appear and mature within weeks.

Biochemistry   Cataract formation in animal models has provided insights into the biochemical mechanisms responsible for the chronic complications of diabetes. Increased activity of the *polyol pathway*, leading to intralenticular accumulation of osmotically active sorbitol and *non-enzymatic glycation* of lens proteins, has been implicated. Drugs (aldose reductase inhibitors and aminoguanidine, respectively) that block these metabolic pathways prevent the development of cataracts in animal models of diabetes.

Treatment   Surgical extraction with implantation of an intra-ocular lens is now a routine procedure.

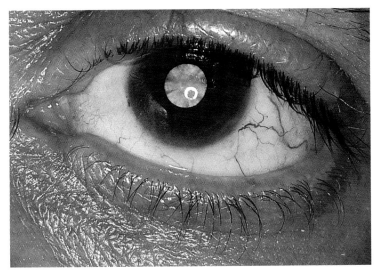

Fig. 76 Cataracts cause loss of the red retinal reflex on direct opthalmoscopy.

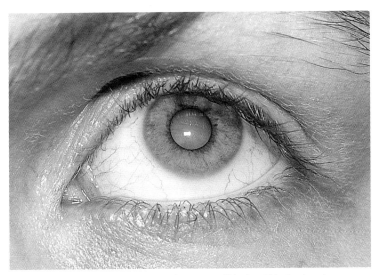

Fig. 77 Acute dense 'snowflake' cataract in a young diabetic which developed over several weeks.

21 / Diabetic neuropathy

Epidemiology and pathogenesis

Peripheral neuropathy is a common complication of diabetes and causes considerable morbidity. Nerve conduction studies are often abnormal at diagnosis of diabetes and tend to improve with control of glycaemia; overactivity of the polyol pathway (p. 53) has been implicated. Transient focal neuropathies can occur in hyperosmolar states (Fig. 66, p. 46). Reversible hemiplegia is also a recognized association of hypoglycaemia (p. 37).

Clinical classification

- Focal neuropathies.
- Distal symmetrical polyneuropathy.
- Motor neuropathies.
- Autonomic neuropathy.

Clinical features

Focal neuropathies may affect cranial nerves, e.g. the oculomotor nerve (Fig. 66, p. 46), or peripheral nerves, e.g. median, common peroneal nerves (Fig. 128, p. 86); these probably represent localized vascular lesions. Spontaneous recovery is the rule. Motor neuropathies (Fig. 78) include painful amyotrophy (Fig. 79) which may cause constitutional disturbance with weight loss ('neuropathic cachexia'). Chronic symmetrical neuropathy may be asymptomatic. Symptoms include paraesthesiae, numbness and pain (particularly nocturnal). Signs of neuropathy (absent ankle jerks, diminished vibration sense, dilated veins) may be evident. Denervation of intrinsic foot muscles produces 'clawing' of the toes, thereby exposing the metatarsal heads and predisposing to ulceration (Fig. 80, also see pp. 61–62).

Treatment

Therapeutic options are limited. Glycaemic control should be optimized and appropriate analgesia provided. Tricyclic antidepressants and carbemazepine may alleviate painful symptoms. Reported benefits of aldose reductase inhibitors (see p. 53) have, to date, been unimpressive.

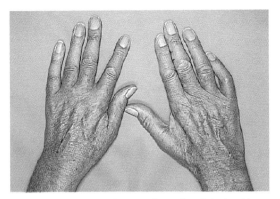

Fig. 78 Marked wasting of the small muscles of the hand in a patient with diabetic polyneuropathy.

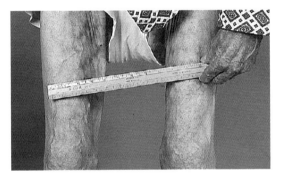

Fig. 79 Diabetic amyotrophy (of Garland) causes painful wasting of the quadriceps muscles.

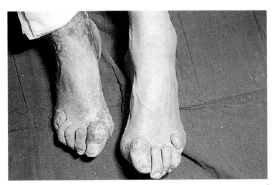

Fig. 80 Chronic sensorimotor polyneuropathy with 'clawing' of toes, callus and dilated veins.

Autonomic neuropathy

Dysfunction of the autonomic nervous system may affect patients with diabetes although it usually remains subclinical. Patients with clinically overt autonomic neuropathy have been found to have a relatively high mortality in follow-up studies.

Clinical features

Erectile impotence. This is the most common manifestation of autonomic neuropathy. Other factors, such as vascular disease, certain drugs (particularly beta-blockers and thiazide diuretics) and psychological factors, are important and require evaluation in impotent patients. Counselling and vacuum condom devices (Fig. 81) or self-administered intracorporeal injections of vasoactive drugs may be helpful.

Postural hypotension. This may be disabling and is difficult to manage. Antihypertensive agents and tricyclics aggravate postural falls in blood pressure; careful use of fludrocortisone may be beneficial.

Gastroparesis. Recurrent vomiting necessitates intravenous fluids. Barium or radionuclide studies reveal delayed gastric emptying (Fig. 82). Metoclopramide and erythromycin may be helpful.

Diarrhoea. This is classically episodic with noctural incontinence. Broad spectrum antibiotics are sometimes of benefit. Other causes of diarrhoea (e.g. gluten-sensitive enteropathy) must be excluded. Malabsorption is not a feature of diabetic diarrhoea.

Bladder paresis. This may produce hesitancy and retention, and predispose to urinary infections.

Gustatory sweats. Rarely, patients may suffer drenching sweats whilst eating (Fig. 83).

Peripheral oedema. Rare; ephedrine may help.

Other features

Arterial calcification. This is common in patients with extensive diabetic neuropathy (Fig. 84).

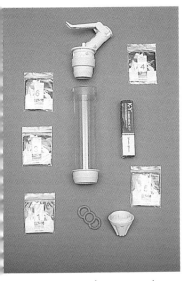

Fig. 81 Components of vacuum condom device for erectile impotence.

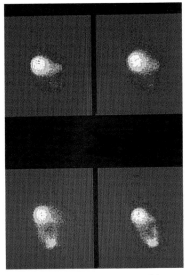

Fig. 82 Sequences from a radionuclide gastric emptying study – $T_{1/2}$ was prolonged to 68 min (normal <20).

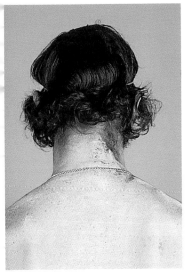

Fig. 83 Gustatory sweating revealed by reaction with iodine powder (brown) on skin.

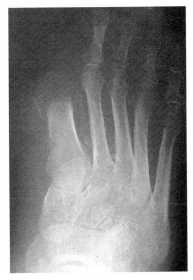

Fig. 84 Arterial calcification in diabetic neuropathy; note amputated hallux.

Autonomic function tests

Subclinical abnormalities of autonomic function are relatively common amongst diabetic patients. These may be detected by simple tests of cardiovascular reflex integrity, e.g. electrocardiographic R–R interval variability during deep breathing, blood pressure response to standing. Computer-aided systems are available which provide comprehensive assessments of autonomic function (Fig. 85). More sensitive assessments may be made using techniques such as the acetylcholine sweatspot test (Fig. 86) and pupillary adaptation to dark.

Prognosis of autonomic neuropathy

Autonomic dysfunction has been implicated in the sudden death of diabetic patients peri-operatively. The mechanism is uncertain although cardiorespiratory arrest has been postulated.

Relation to glycaemic control

Improvements in glycaemic control have little benefical effect on symptomatic autonomic neuropathy, since advanced histological changes (axonal loss, demyelination, obliteration of vasa nervorum; Fig. 87) within nerves are likely to be only partially reversible. Restoration of normoglycaemia by pancreatic transplantation (p. 65) possibly reduces mortality in patients with impaired cardiovascular reflex tests (p. 65), although this has not been confirmed by randomized trials. Patients with insulin-dependent diabetes assigned to intensive glycaemic control in the Diabetic Control and Complications Trial developed fewer abnormal tests of autonomic function tests when assessed after 5 years, although the incidence of clinically overt autonomic dysfunction in these patients was very low.

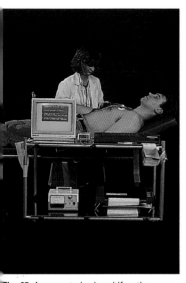

Fig. 85 A computerized multifunction autonomic function test cart.

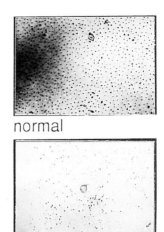

normal

patient (L) foot

Fig. 86 Responses to the acetylcholine sweatspot test (dots indicate innervated glands). A = normal, B = patient.

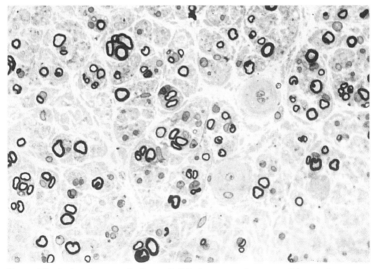

Fig. 87 Histological features of advanced diabetic neuropathy – axonal loss and demyelination.

22 / The diabetic foot

The syndrome of diabetic foot disease incorporates elements of peripheral and autonomic neuropathy, peripheral vascular disease and secondary infection. Diabetic patients have a 10- to 20-fold increased risk of non-traumatic amputation compared with the non-diabetic population (Fig. 58, p. 42). Foot disease is therefore an important cause of morbidity in diabetic patients.

The neuropathic diabetic foot

This is insensitive (due to sensory neuropathy), dry (due to sympathetic denervation) and warm (well-perfused in the absence of coexisting peripheral vascular disease). Areas of high pressure develop due to alterations in foot anatomy that occur as a result of denervation of intrinsic foot muscles (Fig. 80, p. 56). Calluses develop over these areas (Fig. 88). Shearing forces during walking cause disruption of the underlying tissues which may lead to ulceration, secondary infection and gangrene (Fig. 89). Management involves bed rest, antibiotics and judicious surgery.

Charcot neuroarthropathy

Increased blood flow through the foot, together with abnormal loading, may cause fractures with minimal trauma (Fig. 115, p. 78). The foot may be warm, tender and swollen, leading to an erroneous diagnosis of infection. Further fractures cause progressive disorganization of the fore-, mid- and hindfoot (Fig. 116, p. 78), leading eventually to a deformed neuro-arthopathic foot which is at high risk of ulceration (Fig. 90). Treatment during the acute stages usually involves immobilization, e.g. in a 'walking' plaster or removable cast (Fig. 91). Recently, bisphosphonates have been used with the aim of suppressing bone remodelling. Surgical footware subsequently helps to prevent ulceration.

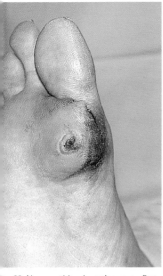

Fig. 88 Neuropathic ulceration over first metatarsal head – note callus formation.

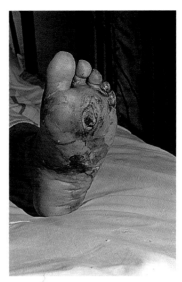

Fig. 89 Limb-threatening deep tissue infection with neuropathic ulcer as portal of entry.

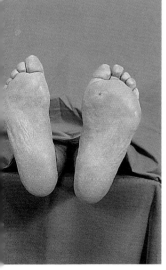

Fig. 90 End-stage Charcot neuro-arthropathy – foot deformity predisposes ulceration.

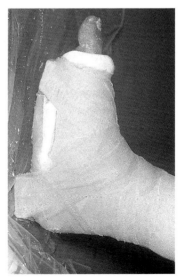

Fig. 91 A 'walking' plaster cast may facilitate healing of ulcers.

23 / **Diabetic nephropathy**

Incidence Approximately 30% of diabetic patients develop nephropathy (Fig. 92). In the UK, approximately 600 diabetic patients per annum develop end-stage renal failure. The incidence amongst non-insulin-dependent patients is ~20% although black and south-Asian patients appear to be at higher risk than white Europeans.

Diagnosis and clinical course Proteinuria is the hallmark of diabetic nephropathy. Initially, urinary albumin excretion is between 30 and 300 mg/day (so-called 'microalbuminuria') and sensitive radioimmunoassays are required to quantify proteinuria; an early morning urinary albumin: creatinine ratio is an alternative. When albumin excretion exceeds 300 mg/day, the Albustix® test becomes positive. Nephrotic syndrome may develop (Fig. 93). Blood pressure rises, although initially it remains within the normotensive range. Glomerular filtration declines with progression to end-stage renal failure over 7–10 years (although with considerable interindividual variation). Morbidity and mortality from coronary heart and peripheral vascular disease are high. Renal biopsy is usually unnecessary unless there are atypical features, particularly a rapid deterioration in renal function or absence of retinopathy.

Management Strict glycaemic control reduces the incidence of microalbuminuria but has no effect in the later stages of nephropathy. Control of hypertension is essential; cigarette smoking should be avoided. Angiotensin-converting enzyme inhibitors have a renoprotective effect even in normotensive patients. Protein restriction is usually recommended. Dialysis eventually becomes necessary (Fig. 2, p. 2, and Fig. 94); renal transplantation is the treatment of choice (Fig. 95). Although advanced retinopathy is common, visual impairment is not a contraindication to renal replacement therapy.

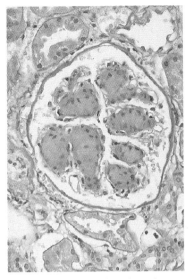

Fig. 92 Diabetic glomerulonephropathy with eosinophilic nodular Kimmelstiel-Wilson lesions.

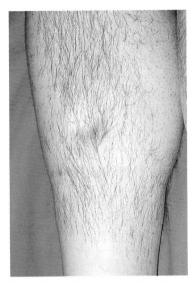

Fig. 93 Nephrotic syndrome, with pitting oedema, due to diabetic glomerulosclerosis.

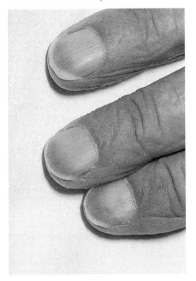

Fig. 94 Changes in nail colour (brown line) are a characteristic feature of chronic renal failure.

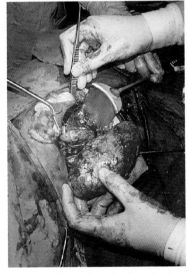

Fig. 95 Renal transplantation (usually after a period of dialysis) is the treatment of choice.

24 / Pancreas and islet transplantation

Pancreatic transplantation

This was first performed in the 1960s. Subsequent advances in surgical techniques and immunosuppression have stimulated interest in the procedure, and by 1995 more than 6500 pancreas transplants had been performed worldwide in selected patients with insulin-dependent diabetes mellitus. In most instances, pancreas transplantation is performed in patients with renal failure secondary to diabetic nephropathy. Since these patients will usually receive a kidney transplant (Fig. 95, p. 64), the dilemma of potentially hazardous immunosuppressive drug therapy is immaterial. The ethical issues of pancreas transplantation in patients without end-stage renal failure are more complex, although some patients have received solitary pancreas transplants. The donor organ is usually cadaveric.

Effects of a pancreas transplant

Metabolic effects of successful pancreatic transplantation include:
- freedom from insulin injections
- normalization of glycated haemoglobin levels
- no risk of severe hypoglycaemia.

The beneficial effects of pancreatic transplantation on chronic microvascular and neurological complications have in general been limited, reflecting the advanced stage of complications by the time of transplantation. A pancreas graft may protect a transplanted kidney from the redevelopment of diabetic nephropathy.

Islet cell transplantation

This technique is under development and is still regarded as experimental (Figs 96–98). Although a few patients have been rendered insulin-independent for 12 months or more, major technical difficulties remain to be overcome. Problems of purification and immunogenicity are research priorities.

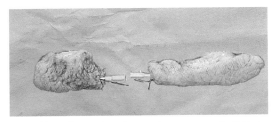

Fig. 96 Islet cell transplantation – a donor pancreas is divided and perfused with collagenase.

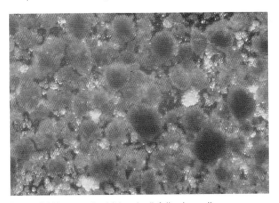

Fig. 97 Dithizone-stained islets (red) following collagenase digestion of the pancreas.

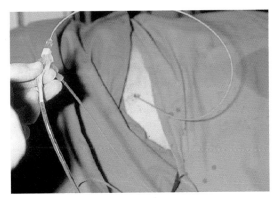

Fig. 98 Purified islets are infused into the portal system under local anaesthesia.

25 / Hypertension and diabetes mellitus

Non-insulin-dependent diabetes

Hypertension (Fig. 99) is commonly associated with non-insulin-dependent diabetes and contributes to mortality from coronary heart disease (p. 71), stroke (Fig. 100) and other complications (Fig. 101). The prevalence approaches 50%, with Afro-Caribbean patients being at particular risk. Hypertension is associated with insulin resistance (p. 25) and it has been hypothesized that the two conditions may be causally related. Drug therapy with beta-blockers and high-dose thiazide diuretics aggravates insulin resistance (p. 23). While the clinical significance of this effect is uncertain, treatment with these agents has not produced the expected reduction in mortality from coronary heart disease. Adverse effects of these agents on plasma lipids (increased very low density lipoproteins and hypercholesterolaemia, respectively; see p. 69) have been suggested as a possible explanation. Associated haemostatic abnormalities (increased fibrinogen and factor VII, reduced activity of plasminogen activator inhibitor-1) may contribute to atherogenesis. Angiotensin-converting enzymes inhibitors and alpha-blockers improve insulin action.

Insulin-dependent diabetes

Hypertension is particularly associated with diabetic nephropathy (p. 63) and plays an important role in determining the rate of decline of renal function. Degrees of hypertension below World Health Organization diagnostic criteria (160/95) may be clinically important. Impairment of the physiological fall in blood pressure that occurs during the night may also be significant. Nephropathy is more prevalent among patients who have hypertensive parents, suggesting that hypertension may be an inherited factor which increases the risk of renal disease.

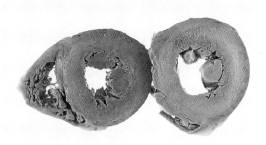

Fig. 99 Postmortem pathology sections showing concentric left ventricular hypertrophy.

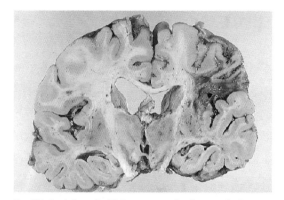

Fig. 100 Healed cerebral infarct – mortality from stroke is increased in diabetic patients.

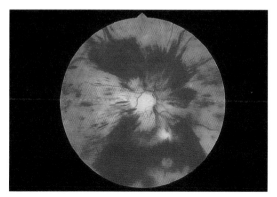

Fig. 101 Central retinal vein thrombosis in a hypertensive diabetic patient.

26 / Lipid metabolism and diabetes mellitus

Diabetes is associated with quantitative and qualitative alterations in plasma lipids which increase the risk of atheromatous complications, particularly coronary heart disease (see p. 71).

Non-insulin-dependent diabetes

The most common abnormalities of plasma lipids are elevated low-density lipoprotein (LDL) cholesterol and triglyceride concentrations in concert with low high-density lipoprotein (HDL) cholesterol levels. Hypertriglyceridaemia may reflect an increased supply of non-esterified fatty acids to the liver in conjunction with elevated portal insulin levels. Primary hyperlipidaemias may coexist with diabetes mellitus (Figs 102 and 103).

Treatment Treatment involves dietary measures, optimization of glycaemic control (insulin stimulates tissue LDL receptor activity and glycation of LDL particles may impair their clearance) and, if these measures prove inadequate, specific lipid-lowering drugs. The fibrates are the agents of choice. Glycaemic control may also be improved to a modest degree by lowering plasma fatty acid levels, thereby reducing the activity of the glucose–fatty acid (Randle) cycle.

Insulin-dependent diabetes

Patients with good glycaemic control usually have relatively normal plasma lipid profiles. Acute metabolic decompensation may be associated with marked hyperlipidaemia (Figs 104 and 105). This resolves with insulin therapy, in part reflecting the effect of insulin on the endothelial enzyme lipoprotein lipase which hydrolyses circulating triglycerides. The rare syndromes of lipoatrophy (see pp. 25 and 26) may be associated with marked hyperlipidaemia.

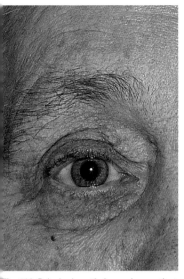

Fig. 102 Palpebral xanthelasma in a patient with diabetes and hypercholesterolaemia.

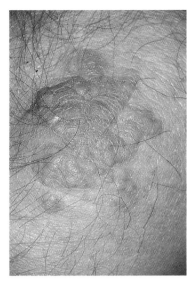

Fig. 103 Tuberose xanthomata in a diabetic patient (Fredrickson type III hyperlipoproteinaemia).

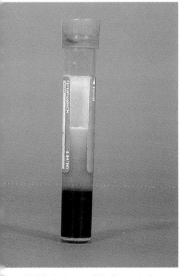

Fig. 104 Marked reversible lipaemia in an insulin-dependent patient with diabetic ketoacidosis.

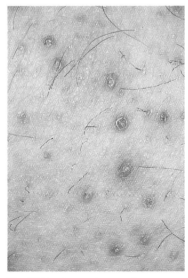

Fig. 105 Eruptive xanthomata due to marked hypertriglyceridaemia in non-insulin-dependent diabetes.

27 / **Coronary heart disease**

Mortality rates

Coronary heart disease is the most common cause o mortality among diabetic patients. It is the major cause of death in patients over 40 years of age and i patients with disease duration exceeding 30 years. Patients with proteinuria are at greatly increased risk of atheromatous cardiovascular disease (see p. 63). Diabetes is a major risk factor for coronary heart disease and negates the usual relative protectio conferred to premenopausal women.

Risk factors

Other risk factors for atherosclerosis in diabetic patients are:

- hypertension
- hyperlipidaemia
- positive family history of atheroma
- cigarette smoking.

Modifiable risk factors should be sought and corrected wherever possible.

Pathology

The pathology of coronary heart disease in diabetic patients does not differ from that in the non-diabeti population (Fig. 106). A specific diabetic cardiomyopathy has been postulated which may contribute to the development of cardiac failure in some patients (Fig. 107).

Acute myocardial infarction

The mortality rate of patients with diabetes followin myocardial infarction is higher than that for non-diabetic subjects with similar-sized infarcts, eve with thrombolytic therapy (Fig. 4, p. 2). Glycaemic control is important and intravenous insulin infusion have been shown to be effective in the management of diabetic patients on coronary care units. Metform should be avoided in patients with overt ischaemic heart disease or cardiac failure (see p. 31). Seconda preventative measures should be considered.

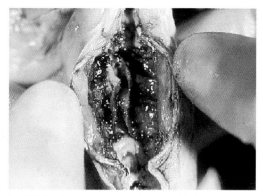

Fig. 106 Fatal coronary artery atheroma with thrombus formation leading to myocardial infarction.

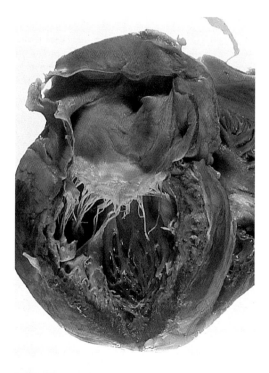

Fig. 107 Dilated left ventricle from patient with ischaemic heart disease and heart failure.

28 / **Peripheral vascular disease**

Together with neuropathy and infection, peripheral vascular disease contributes to foot disease in patients with diabetes (see p. 61). The incidence of peripheral vascular disease is increased approximately twofold in diabetic patients. Abnormalities of circulating lipids, hypertension and smoking are recognized risk factors for peripheral vascular disease. The role of hyperinsulinaemia *per se* remains controversial.

Clinical features

Patients are asymptomatic until significant arterial stenoses develop. Symptoms may then include:

- intermittent claudication
- rest pain with critical ischaemia (Fig. 108)
- ischaemic ulceration – this accounts for only approximately 10% of diabetic foot ulcers, but coexisting vascular disease may impede healing of ulcers that are predominantly of neuropathic origin, particularly when there is superadded infection in soft tissues or bone.

Assessment

Clinical evaluation includes palpation of peripheral pulses and auscultation for bruits. Trophic changes in the skin are sought and limb temperature is assessed. Risk factors for atherosclerosis and any aggravating disorders (e.g. anaemia) should be sought. Doppler studies are performed (Fig. 109) prior to angiographic evaluation of the site and extent of the lesions which often affect the distal arterial tree.

Management

Foot care is of great importance and patients should receive appropriate instruction. Timely chiropody may avert more serious lesions. Reconstructive surgery or angioplasty may preserve limbs although major amputation is still sometimes the only option (Fig. 110 and Fig. 58, p. 42).

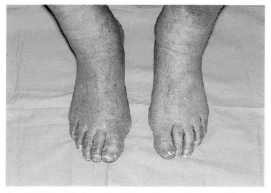

Fig. 108 Critical ischaemia of the patient's right foot with rest pain – Buerger's sign is positive.

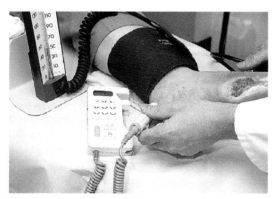

Fig. 109 Measurement of blood pressure and arterial flow using a Doppler probe.

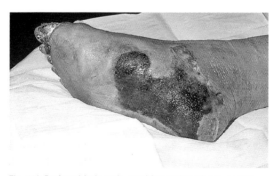

Fig. 110 Profound ischaemia requiring major (above- or below-knee) amputation.

29 / Skin disease and diabetes mellitus

The skin of diabetic patients may be affected by:
- Lesions that are virtually specific to diabetes.
- Lesions associated with aspects of the diabetic syndrome (e.g. insulin resistance).
- Lesions associated with diabetic complications.
- Skin disorders that also occur in non-diabetics but which are more frequently seen amongst diabetics.

Necrobiosis lipoidica diabeticorum

This uncommon lesion (Fig. 111) is closely associated with diabetes, although it may sometimes pre-date the development of glucose intolerance. The lesions typically affect the pre-tibial skin but may develop at sites of trauma. Treatment with topical steroids, skin grafts or cryotherapy is often unsatisfactory.

Vitiligo

This is a marker of autoimmunity (Fig. 112). Other autoimmune diseases, e.g. Graves' disease, (Fig. 26, p. 20) and pernicious anaemia, are more common in insulin-dependent diabetics.

Bullae

Rarely, bullae may occur in patients with neuropathy, probably reflecting unrecognized trauma (Fig. 113).

Diabetic dermopathy

This appears as red/brown papules on the shins (Fig. 114) which progress to shiny hyperpigmented or scaly scars. Trauma and neuropathy may be factors in its pathogenesis.

Granuloma annulare

This occurs in non-diabetics and it is uncertain whether there is more than just a chance association with diabetes.

Other lesions

Acanthosis nigricans (Fig. 38, p. 26) and allergic reactions to therapy (Fig. 45, p. 30; Figs 49 and 50, p. 34) are uncommon.

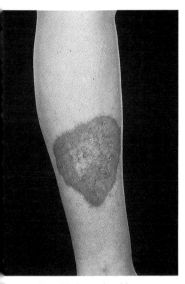

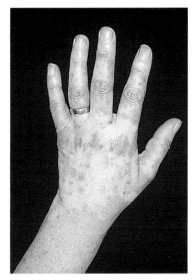

Fig. 111 Necrobiosis on the shin, comprising plaques with surface telangiectasia and yellowish centre.

Fig. 112 Vitiligo is a skin marker in autoimmune disease such as insulin-dependent diabetes.

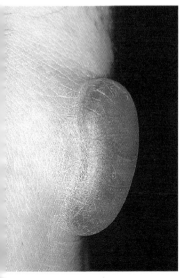

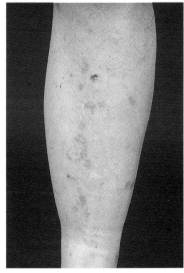

Fig. 113 Tense bulla on foot in a patient with diabetic peripheral neuropathy.

Fig. 114 Diabetic dermopathy on shin.

Osteopenia and fractures

Patients with insulin-dependent diabetes of long duration have reduced bone mineral densities compared with the non-diabetic population. The clinical significance of this is uncertain, since fractures other than those of the metatarsal bones in neuropathic patients (Fig. 115) are uncommon.

Localized osteopenia

This appears to be of importance in the pathogenesis of Charcot neuro-arthropathy (Fig. 116; see also p. 61). Increased blood flow through the neuropathic foot may be an important contributory factor.

Limited joint mobility

Diabetes of long duration may result in thickening of the subcutaneous tissues, producing limited mobility and stiffness around joints. The 'prayer' sign may be elicited (Fig. 117). In addition, the skin of affected patients may have a waxy appearance reminiscent of scleroderma.

Capsulitis

Adhesive capsulitis of the shoulder (and sometimes hips) appears to be associated with diabetes and may differ histologically from the idiopathic forms of these conditions.

Gout

An increased serum uric acid concentration is a marker for coronary heart disease and is associated with glucose intolerance (Fig. 118). Hyperuricaemia is also more prevalent amongst individuals with obesity, hyperlipidaemia and hypertension (see p. 25). In non-diabetic individuals, plasma uric acid concentrations are inversely related to rates of insulin-mediated glucose disposal, as determined using the glucose 'clamp' technique (Fig. 36, p. 24).

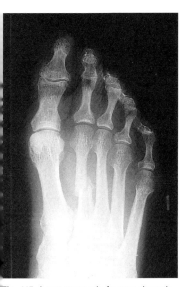

Fig. 115 A non-traumatic fracture through the shaft of the second metatarsal in a patient with severe neuropathy.

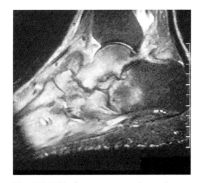

Fig. 116 MRI of acute neuroarthropathy showing extensive bone destruction and tissue inflammation (high signal).

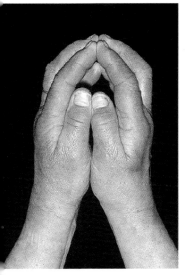

Fig. 117 Limited joint mobility with a positive 'prayer' sign in an insulin-dependent patient.

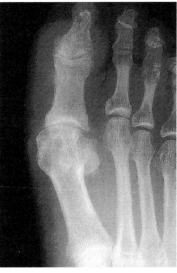

Fig. 118 Gout with secondary osteoarthitis affecting the first metatarsophalangeal joint.

31 / Infection and diabetes mellitus

Fungal and bacterial infections

Although these infections (Figs 119 and 120) may be encountered more frequently in diabetic patients, it remains uncertain whether the overall risk of infection is increased. Diabetes is considered to be a risk factor for pulmonary tuberculosis. Recurrent cutaneous or urogenital infections, e.g. vulvo-vaginal candidiasis (Fig. 120) or balanitis, may be the presenting feature of diabetes, and their occurrence should prompt appropriate investigations (see p. 9).

Predisposing factors

Physical factors. Severe invasive infections may develop because of particular predisposing factors that arise from the diabetic state. For example, chronic complications such as foot ulcers provide portals of entry for microorganisms to soft tissues (Fig. 89, p. 62) and bone. Polymicrobial infections with streptococci, staphylococci and anaerobes are usual. Autonomic neuropathy (see p. 57) predisposes to urinary stasis and ascending infections (Fig. 121).

Metabolic factors. The ability of neutrophil leucocytes to migrate, ingest and kill organisms is compromised by hyperglycaemia. In turn, infections may lead to a deterioration in metabolic control; infections are the most common identifiable precipitating causes of diabetic ketoacidosis (Fig. 61, p. 44). Metabolic control is important in the management of infections in diabetic patients; the association between the rare, serious condition of rhinocerebral mucormycosis (Fig. 122) and diabetic ketoacidosis is particularly noteworthy.

Viral infections

Viral infections have been implicated in the aetiology of insulin-dependent diabetes (p. 11).

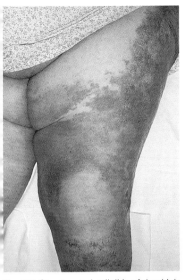

Fig. 119 Streptococcal cellulitis of the thigh leading to deterioration in glycaemic control.

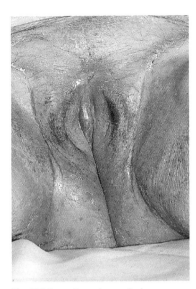

Fig. 120 Extensive vulvo-vaginal candidiasis.

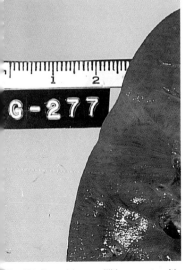

Fig. 121 Necrotizing papillitis presents with fever and colic – note sloughed renal papilla.

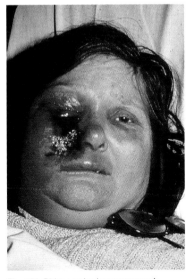

Fig. 122 Rhinocerebral mucormycosis – enucleation of the eye was necessary despite antifungal therapy.

32 / Diabetes mellitus and pregnancy

Effects on glycaemia
Pregnancy is associated with a deterioration in glycaemic control due to hormone-induced insulin resistance. Insulin requirements therefore increase in insulin-treated patients but fall to pre-pregnancy levels immediately postpartum. Patients treated with diet or tablets may require insulin temporarily. Pre-existing retinopathy and nephropathy may progress during pregnancy.

Gestational diabetes
Diabetes that is first diagnosed during pregnancy is known as 'gestational diabetes'. In the majority of cases, glucose tolerance returns to normal postpartum, although the long-term risk of non-insulin-dependent diabetes is increased. Impaired glucose tolerance (see p. 5) in pregnancy is treated as if it were diabetes.

Outcome of diabetic pregnancy
Perinatal mortality for diabetic pregnancies has reduced considerably, although it remains higher than for non-diabetic pregnancies. The causes of excess perinatal mortality include stillbirth and major congenital malformations. The overall risk of congenital malformations is increased approximately threefold by diabetes (Fig. 123). Maternal glycaemia during fetal organogenesis (between 7 and 10 weeks gestation) is inversely related to the risk of malformations. Pre-pregnancy counselling with attainment of excellent glycaemic control before conception is the ideal. Episodes of hypoglycaemia are not harmful to the fetus, whereas maternal ketoacidosis often results in miscarriage. Pre-eclampsia is more frequent in diabetic mothers.

Effects on the fetus
Fetal macrosomia (Fig. 124) increases the risk of dystocia. Neonatal hypoglycaemia, polycythemia and respiratory distress syndrome are increased and caesarian section rates are higher.

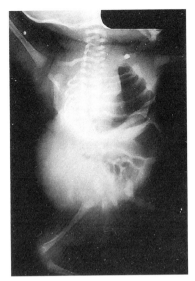

Fig. 123 Sacral agenesis – part of the caudal regression syndrome.

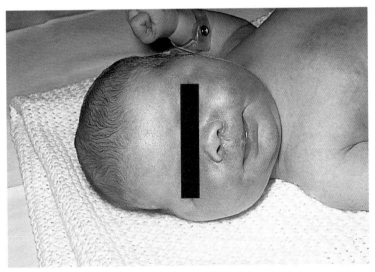

Fig. 124 Neonatal macrosomia and polycythaemia in the infant of a diabetic mother.

33 / Childhood, adolescence and old age

Diabetes in childhood

With rare exceptions, diabetes developing in childhood is insulin-dependent (type 1) diabetes. Diabetes in childhood is compatible with normal schooling and activities, the main metabolic complication being hypoglycaemia (see p. 37). Less frequent is ketoacidosis (see p. 43), although children are especially prone to the serious complication of cerebral oedema during treatment (Fig. 125). Diet and insulin dose are tailored, with the aim of achieving normal physiological development. Clinically overt diabetic complications are uncommon in childhood.

Adolescence

Puberty is associated with an increase in insulin requirements, in part due to physiological insulin resistance. The emotional tensions of adolescence may contribute to eating disorders (e.g. anorexia nervosa), which are more common in young female diabetics. Idiopathic 'brittle' diabetes (recurrent disruptive episodes of ketoacidosis and/or severe hypoglycaemia) due to deliberate manipulation is a behavioural disturbance which often responds poorly to psychotherapy.

Diabetes in the elderly

The aims of treatment may be modified by considerations of life expectancy and concomitant medical conditions. Coexisting cardiovascular and cerebrovascular disease are common. Although the majority of elderly patients have non-insulin-dependent diabetes, insulin therapy is sometimes necessary. Physical and psychological disabilites allied to social isolation pose particular problems (Figs 126 and 127). Avoidance of hypoglycaemia is paramount. Care should also be exercised with sulphonylureas (p. 39).

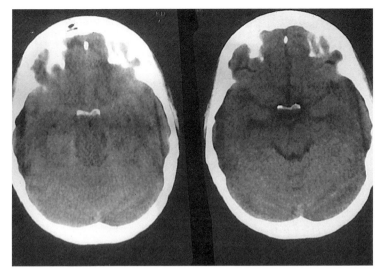

Fig. 125 CT scans of an 11-year-old with ketoacidósis showing cerebral oedema (L) and after recovery (R).

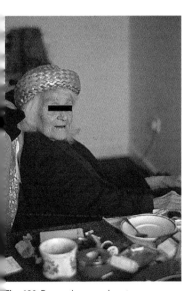

Fig. 126 Dementia secondary to cerebrovascular disease is more prevalent in elderly diabetics.

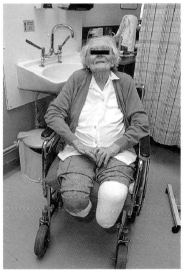

Fig. 127 Elderly patients are also more likely to have associated chronic physical disabilities.

34 / **Social and legal aspects of diabetes mellitus**

Employment for diabetic patients

Iatrogenic hypoglycaemia is the principal concern that limits employment prospects in some professions where this might result in injury to the patient or to others.

Diet- or tablet-treated patients

Patients should encounter few barriers to employment. Employers are encouraged to view potential employees according to their suitability and to be sympathetic to diabetic patients, who in general have good attendance and performance records.

Insulin-treated patients

Insulin-treated patients are barred from entry into the armed forces or police in the UK. They are also excluded from driving passenger-carrying vehicles (see below). Certain occupations (e.g. steeplejack, airline pilot) present obvious risks.

Driving and diabetes

Group 1 licence

In the UK, diabetics are legally required to inform the licensing authority (DVLA) at diagnosis and thereafter if complications develop, e.g. neuropathy (Figs 128 and 130), or if there are important changes in treatment, e.g. starting insulin. Ordinary car or motorbike licences are renewed every 3 years subject to satisfactory medical reports. All insulin-treated drivers must carry glucose tablets (or an alternative) in the car. Symptomatic unawareness of hypoglycaemia (see p. 39) is a particular risk. Retinopathy (pp. 47–52) may impair visual acuity (Fig. 129). In addition, patients who have received extensive laser therapy may have impaired night vision and restricted visual fields.

Group 2 licence

Insulin-treated patients are barred from applying for licences for 'large goods vehicles' or 'passenger-carrying vehicles'.

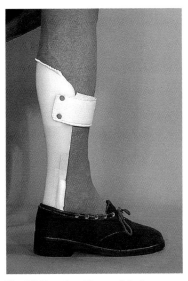

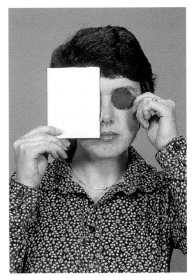

Fig. 128 Foot drop (due to diabetic neuropathy) will prevent normal use of car control pedals.

Fig. 129 Visual acuities are checked for each eye using a pinhole to correct refractive errors.

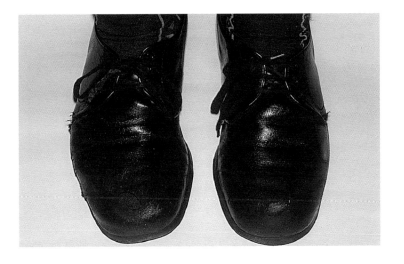

Fig. 130 Severe neuropathy with loss of sensation. Patient has worn through his surgical shoes. Loss of proprioception will also impair pedal control.

35 / **Organization of diabetic care**

Diabetes mellitus is a common and chronic disorder which consumes a significant proportion of the healthcare budget in industrialized countries. Patients require education backed up by readily available expert assistance from a multidisciplinary diabetes care team.

Diabetes centres

Purpose-built diabetes centres have proved to be popular (Fig. 131). Such centres fulfil a multitude of functions:

- Diagnosis and assessment of new patients.
- Long-term follow-up (either for all patients or for selected groups if adequate arrangements exist for the provision or sharing of follow-up with intereste primary care teams).
- Education of patients (and staff).
- Screening for complications (Fig. 132).
- Provision of specialist medical care for special groups (e.g. pregnant diabetics, young patients).

The aim is to provide these services in an accessible and comfortable environment (Fig. 133).

Primary healthcare

The long-term management of diabetic patients in th UK is increasingly being supervised, in whole or in part, in primary care. This approach requires cooperation between hospital-based and primary care to ensure high standards of care.

The role of hospitals

Hospital admission is now rarely required for initiation of insulin therapy but is necessary for the management of acute metabolic emergencies (see pp. 39, 43 and 45). Hospitalization is also frequently required for the management of serious micro- and macrovascular complications, notably foot ulceration (see p. 61).

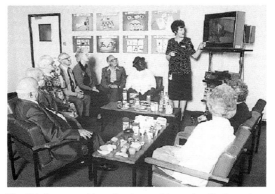

Fig. 131 Group teaching of patients with non-insulin-dependent diabetes in a resource centre.

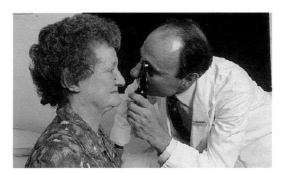

Fig. 132 Annual fundoscopy by trained staff is essential to detect early retinopathy. Retinal photography is an alternative.

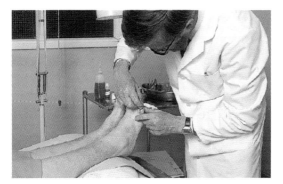

Fig. 133 Diabetes resource centres also house important ancillary services such as chiropody.

Index

Hypoglycaemia (*contd*)
  sulphonylureas and, 39
  symptoms, 37
  unrecognized, 39
Hypopituitarism, 19, 20
Hypotension, postural, 57
Hypothyroidism, primary, 19

Infection and diabetes, 79–80
Insulin
  allergy, 34
  anabolic effects of, 23
  discovery of, 3–4
  resistance, 23, 24, 25, 26
  therapy, 33–4
Insulin-dependent diabetes
  autoimmune markers, 13, 14
  autonomic function tests and, 59
  biochemistry of, 23
  diet and, 27, 28
  employment and, 85
  environmental factors, 11
  epidemiology of, 7, 8
  genetic factors, 11
  hypertension and, 63, 67–8
  lipid metabolism and, 69, 70
  pathophysiology, 11, 12
  presenting features, 13, 14
  retinopathy and, 47
  surgery for, 41, 42
  treatment, 13
Insulinomas, pancreatic, 39, 40
Islet cell transplantation, 65–6

Joint mobility, limited, 77, 78

Karela, 32
Ketoacidosis, diabetic, 43–4, 83, 84
  infection and, 79
  maternal, 81
Ketostix, 35, 43

Laser therapy for retinopathy, 51, 52
Leprechaunism, 25, 26
Lipid metabolism and diabetes, 69–70
Lipoatrophic diabetes, 25, 26, 34

Macrosomia, fetal, 81, 82
Maculopathy, 49, 50
Maternally inherited diabetes, 21
Metabolic control
  infection and, 79
  monitoring, 35–6
Metformin, 31, 32, 41, 71
MODY, 21, 22
Mucormycosis, rhinocerebral, 43, 79, 80
Myocardial infarction, 1, 2, 71
Myotonic dystrophy, 21, 22

Necrobiosis lipoidica diabeticorum, 75, 76
Necrotizing papillitis, 80
Nephropathy, diabetic, 1, 2, 63–4
  hypertension and, 67
Neurodegenerative disorders, 21, 22
Neuropathy, diabetic, 1, 2, 55–60
  autonomic, 57–60
  driving and, 85, 86
  focal, 46
  fractures and, 77, 78
  of foot, 61, 62
Non-insulin dependent diabetes
  biochemistry of, 23
  clinical features, 15
  diet and, 27
  epidemiology, 7, 8
  hypertension and, 67, 68
  lipid metabolism and, 69, 70
  pathogenesis, 15, 16
  retinopathy and, 47
  surgery for, 41, 42

Obesity, 27–8
Organization of diabetic care, 87–8
Osteopenia, 77

Pancreas
  disease of, 17, 18
  transplantation, 65
Pen injectors, 33, 34
Peripheral oedema, 57
Peripheral vascular disease, 73–4
Phaeochromocytoma, 19, 24
Plant remedies, 31, 32
Pneumomediastinum, 43, 44
Polycystic ovary syndrome, 25, 26
Polyol pathway, overactivity of, 53, 55
Pre-eclampsia, 81
Pregnancy and diabetes, 81–2
Primary healthcare, 87
Proteinuria, 63
Pulmonary tuberculosis, 79

Rash, drug, 30
Renal failure, 1, 2, 63–4, 67
Retinopathy, diabetic, 1, 2, 47–52, 63
  classification, 47, 48
  driving and, 85, 86
  screening for, 51, 52, 88
  treatment, 51
Rhinocerebral mucormycosis, 43, 79, 80

Screening for diabetic retinopathy, 51, 52, 88
Secondary diabetes, 17–20
Skeletal and connective tissue disease, 77–8
Skin disease and diabetes, 75–6
Stroke, 45, 67, 68
Sulphonylureas, 29–30, 41, 45, 46, 83
  hypoglycaemia and, 39